Children in Society:
Politics, policies and interventions

Edited by Craig Newnes

PCCS Books
Monmouth

First published 2015

PCCS Books Ltd
Wyastone Business Park
Wyastone Leys
Monmouth
NP25 3SR
UK
Tel +44 (0)1600 891 509
www.pccs-books.co.uk

This collection © Craig Newnes, 2015

The individual chapters © the authors, 2015

All rights reserved.

No part of this publication may be reproduced, stored in a retrieval system, transmitted or utilised in any form by any means, electronic, mechanical, photocopying or recording or otherwise, without permission in writing from the publishers.

The authors have asserted their right to be identified as the authors of this work in accordance with the Copyright, Designs and Patents Act 1988.

Children in Society: Politics, policies and interventions

A CIP catalogue record for this book is available from the British Library.

ISBN 978 1 906254 80 3

Cover designed in the UK by Old Dog Graphics
Typeset in the UK by Raven Books
Printed by Imprint Digital, Exeter, UK

Acknowledgements

I should like to acknowledge the good work of the contributors to this volume and the faith of Heather and Maggie at PCCS Books. Thanks too, to Nick Radcliffe for the kick-start. Without the copy-editing of Kathleen Steeden my own editing would have been so much harder, and without the support of my family, the hours spent in the shed or study would have proven intolerable. So, let's hear it for love.

Dedication

To Alice

Contents

Introduction: Protecting children, projecting childhood   1
Craig Newnes

Part one: Just kids?

1. Children and childhood constructed   7
   Craig Newnes
2. Constructing innocence and risk as a rationale for intervention   33
   Melissa Burkett
3. The Stolen Generations: The forced removal of First Peoples children in Australia   50
   Pat Dudgeon, Carmen Cubillo and Abigail Bray
4. Children and austerity   82
   Carl Harris
5. Single motherhood   102
   Laura Golding
6. Considering the relationship between vulnerability and child sexual exploitation   122
   Adele Gladman

Part two: Just services?

7. The rights of parents and children in regard to children receiving psychiatric diagnoses and drugs   145
   Peter R. Breggin
8. 'Learning-disabled children'   162
   Katherine Runswick-Cole and Dan Goodley
9. Children and electroconvulsive therapy   181
   Craig Newnes
10. Looking after children: Love, meaning and connection   203
    Carolyn McQueen
11. Don't blame the parents: Is it possible to develop non-blaming models of parental causation of distress?   212
    Rudi Dallos
12. The children's disability living allowance form: Policing dependency with a boundary object   231
    Orly Klein and Carl Walker

About the contributors   247
Name Index   251
Subject Index   254

Introduction
Protecting children, projecting childhood

Craig Newnes

Ten years can seem like the blink of an eye or a long time. Stars that (we are told) burned out millions of years ago continue to glow. Some of the world's children would have done well to have spent five years witnessing those same stars. For many, half a decade is a lifetime; for the majority caught up in the civil war raging in the Democratic Republic of the Congo, five years is the *most* they might expect (see Chapter 1). The privileged of the world might reach an age where five or even ten years doesn't seem so long. I guess I fall into that category.

It is ten years since Nick Radcliffe and I edited *Making and Breaking Children's Lives*.[1] In that time I have become a grandfather, retired from my role as Director of Psychological Therapies in the NHS in Shropshire, lost my dad, attended the funerals of too many close friends, lived on and off in France, and been the songwriter, rhythm guitarist and vocalist for no less than four bands. Somewhere in the mix I moved house (gaining a greenhouse, pond and goat-shed in the process – ha!), watched my various children move from primary to secondary school or to university and postgraduate education, spent a fortune on school shoes, and published a volume critiquing the profession of clinical psychology and a second critiquing pretty much the entire Psy industry.[2]

But in the wider world of children and child services? *Making and Breaking Children's Lives* critically examined the nature of childhood, a history of child abuse, domestic violence and the discourse of responsibility as applied to young people. Four chapters were devoted to the inexorable, drug-company-sponsored rise of ADHD inscription.

A third of the volume was devoted to attempts by professionals to create better futures for children.

Ten years on it would be difficult – unaided by drugs – to feel sanguine about the current state of childhood and children's services. The current volume informs us that in those ten years some 30,000 US citizens have been *shot* (often accidentally) by *children under six* (see Chapter 1); children under 14 are at risk of electrocution (termed electroconvulsive therapy) in Australia, China and several US states, and, in Turkey, some as young as nine are given ECT explicitly as a form of torture (see Chapter 9).

Inscription of children as disordered (perhaps 'disordering' would be more accurate, though still individualised) continues as bipolar disorder competes with ADHD for ascendency. The drugging of children marked in these ways is ubiquitous and potentially lethal (see Chapter 7). Article 6 of the UN Convention on the Rights of the Child states 'Children have the right to live.' Of the world's 195 nations, only the United States has yet to ratify the convention; Somalia is in the process of so doing at time of writing.

In the UK there are weekly revelations concerning historical sexual assaults on children by previously feted celebrities and politicians. In the last case we await the unearthing of some 'lost' files, files it is claimed that detail the deaths of assaulted children.

The role of many services – despite the best efforts of certain staff – continues to be one of inscription and assault in the name of treatment. Children are diagnosed by families, teachers, professionals and each other before embarking on careers as Psy recipients. For the majority a drug regimen remains the first response (see Chapter 7). As Grace Jackson noted in her chapter in *Making and Breaking Children's Lives*, the ingestion of psychiatric drugs by the young is a gateway to more drugs – prescribed and illicit – in later life.[3]

Over half this volume concerns efforts by policy makers and Psy professionals to change lives a little for children, at least in the UK, the US and Australia. All are marked by the sheer amount of effort the practitioners put into their work. Most of the authors are parents, some grandparents; all of us are children. Contributors explore the meaning of childhood and the tropes surrounding the concept – from 'vulnerability' to 'sexualised' and 'disabled'. Chapters examine the roles of parents and foster-parents in providing safer environments for children. Authors discuss the willingness of parents – sometimes against financial odds or the mistrust of professionals – to make the family home, with all its messiness, a place where children can feel safe and, dare I say it, love.

Some chapters didn't make it this time despite the authors' best intentions. Chapters on the oppressed lives of children in Palestine, the family court system and the ambiguous position of boarding school education await a third volume, perhaps in another ten years? Imagine – 2025. There are few signs that the world will be a better place for the majority. And for children? If the authors of this volume are anything to go by, then perhaps.

Endnotes

1. Newnes, C. & Radcliffe, N. (Eds) (2005). *Making and Breaking Children's Lives*. Ross-on-Wye: PCCS Books.
2. Newnes, C. (2014). *Clinical Psychology: A critical examination*. Ross-on-Wye: PCCS Books; Newnes, C. (2015). *Inscription, Diagnosis and Deception in the Mental Health Industry: How Psy governs us all*. Basingstoke: Palgrave Macmillan.
3. Jackson, G. (2005). Cybernetic children: How technologies change and constrain the developing mind. In. C. Newnes and N. Radcliffe (Eds). *Making and Breaking Children's Lives* (pp. 90–104). Ross-on-Wye: PCCS Books.

Part one
Just kids?

Chapter 1
Children and childhood constructed

Craig Newnes

At eight I had my first summer job. Living in Hopton-on-Sea on the border of Suffolk and Norfolk made summer work easy to find as there were several holiday camps some distance from the railway station. Holidaymakers needed both help with their luggage and directions to their destinations. Directions were freely offered but luggage was carted on home-constructed wooden barrows; hence our title: 'barrow-boys' (or 'barrerbouys' in the vernacular). We were old enough to push a low cart laden with suitcases but not sufficiently versed in notions of the market to negotiate our rate of pay for each journey. There were up to ten trips every Saturday, the longest being about five miles. The reward was left to the generosity of our customers (a habit I have yet to break). Some, frequently Americans, would pay up to a pound sterling (a small fortune in 1963) for even short trips, while others would grudgingly part with a tanner (the equivalent of two-and-a-half-pence) for the 40-minute trek to the 'Ponderosa'. Were we exploited? Were we children or workers at weekends? Perhaps we were service providers.

It may seem obvious to the reader what is meant by children and childhood. Any experience of child and adolescent mental health services, however, will have revealed a degree of ambiguity. In the UK NHS different regions and health administrative structures differ in their definitions of the points at which a child becomes an adolescent and then an adult. For some the definitions depend on education: a child becomes an adolescent when she enters secondary education, becoming an adult when she leaves the school system. For others there are age demarcations: 'children' remain children until age 13 and are adolescents until age 20. In other words, adolescents are teenagers. For others 'children' effectively become 'adults' if child services cannot cope; nineteenth-century US asylums had so many children behind their walls that a new discipline of inpatient child psychiatry began by default. In the middle of the nineteenth century Bellevue Asylum in New York held over 1,000 children under the age of 16.[1]

Beyond the confines of structuralised service definitions, for many parents their children remain 'children' all their lives. Talk to someone in his eighties on a bus about his 'kids' and you will soon discover they are in their fifties or sixties. For parents whose offspring never leave home or, due to being marked as 'disabled' have been institutionalised, the social context re-languages the child as 'lazy', 'dependent', or, in the case of those with physical disabilities or psychiatric diagnoses, 'eternal children' or 'tragic'.[2] Service definitions of childhood reflect wider societal ambiguities; in the UK a 10-year-old can be tried for murder, but that same child would have to wait until 16 to legally begin a sexual relationship, 17 to drive, 18 to vote, etc. In the USA, the age demarcation lines differ between states for driving, owning a gun and buying alcohol. The last example is further complicated in the UK where many stores now demand that a person buying alcohol looks 25 even though the legal qualification is 18. Once a person has been asked for proof of age, the person at the till cannot serve him or her alcohol unless proof is available in the form of a driving licence or similar; so a 23-year-old without proof of identity will still not be served.

Mothers may have children by age 12 in some parts of India, and in Africa may, aged seven, be looking after the remnants of a family devastated by AIDS. In the US young people carry hand guns; 138,490 Americans were shot by children under six in the decade 1983–1993.[3] Chinese children may work in sweatshops from dawn to dusk. The so-called radicalisation of teenagers finds people younger than 15 blowing themselves and others to pieces in the name of religion or freedom. Involvement in armed struggle has been a feature of childhood in the UK for centuries – boys aged 15 and younger lied about their age to join the navy in the First World War.

This chapter will examine some myths surrounding fluctuating, culturally located notions of childhood. Some attempt will be made to place these myths and associated tropes in historical context before examining ways in which inscriptions of 'abnormality' lead to Psy involvement with children.

Childhood as myth

It is tempting to suggest that 'childhood' is entirely mythic.[4] It is a phase of life open to a wide range of tropes serving the interests of the observer.

'Innocence' and 'vulnerability' are used as descriptors of a period seen as requiring protection, while 'naivety' or 'ignorance' may be offered as rationales for 'education'. In the UK there is considerable hand-wringing over the nature of sex education for primary school children. Lessons concerning sexual relationships can be embedded in a series of talks about 'responsibility' or 'values' or subject to protest from parents who do not want children to be exposed to teaching on sex outside the home (or, sometimes, at all). For some, this parental or religious position can be part of a 'fetishistic glorification of the "innate innocence" of childhood'.[5] Innocence is a trope commonly used in the press – particularly in reports of sexual assault of children – and may be felt as an accurate depiction of life before assault for some victims.

Children are a rich source of literary material, frequently as part of a moralising praxis that, as a narrative, can come to symbolise an age and its approach to the young. Cronos ate all his newborn children until the birth of Zeus, Romulus and Remus were abandoned by their father Amulius to die in the Tiber, and Herod killed all the male children of Jews in his hunt for the baby Jesus. Hansel and Gretel were followed by the *Water Babies* into the consciousness of Victorian England. The pipe-smoking Huck Finn duly made his entrance. In 2015, following a request from the local education council, titles including *The Adventures of Tom Sawyer* and *Thumbelina* were taken off the shelves in the village of Kharbatovo, in the southern Irkutsk Region of Russia. The action was legitimised by a 2012 law aimed at 'protecting children from information that harms their health and development'. The law introduced age restrictions for books, films and theatre productions, among other measures. The council feared that Twain's book might encourage children to become vagrants, and other tales could 'promote disrespect for parents and family values'.[6] It is not clear what reaction the council feared from widespread reading of *Thumbelina* – young local girls marrying toads or moles, perhaps?

An inevitable feature of censorship and control of this type is that those in positions of socially sanctioned power impose their reading of any given text before ruling on its 'suitability' for children and young people. This can produce some striking anomalies; advertisements in the early years of this century featuring a pockmarked and very thin heroin addict, for example, were shown to *increase* heroin use amongst teenagers in areas close to the billboards, an unfortunate consequence of the addict being underweight and good-looking in a dolefully appealing way.

From *Little Dorrit* to *David Copperfield* via Tiny Tim, Dickens invented childhood icons symbolising courage, sanctity or whatever would keep his readership enthralled. *Little Women*, *Peter Pan* and *Just William* remain best sellers, though *Billy Bunter* seems to have lost his following. Perhaps Bunter was never iconic enough – just a greedy public schoolboy getting his just desserts. For some, a UK childhood still mirrors a little of Bunter's boarding school experiences. For the majority of school-age children, the Education Acts of the nineteenth and twentieth centuries ensured access to primary and secondary state education. Other parents prefer to remove children from both systems and there is a long history of the preference for home tuition; Ludwig Wittgenstein, for example, was educated at home until he was 14. Perhaps a less successful example is the 12-year-old son of Agrippina, home tutored by no less a teacher than Seneca. The 12-year-old grew up to become the Emperor Nero.

The moralising nature of childhood myth-making is clear in early-readers' series *Janet and John* and it appears in more specific form in several 'instructional' tales targeted at children inscribed with bipolar disorder. *My Bipolar Roller Coaster Feelings* and *Brandon and the Bipolar Bear* both end with the somewhat wayward heroes being 'sorted out' with medication.[7]

Children also have their place within superstition and myth. In Durham and the north of England a centuries-old myth claims that stepping over a child's head will stunt the child's growth: 'the overleapt infant would never grow'.[8] In families children are mythologised from birth. A child born with, say, bright blue eyes may be immediately declared to be 'just like Aunt Grace or Uncle Jack', a positioning that may recur if Grace or Jack have reputations within the family for particular conduct. A child who is particularly rambunctious in a family context where the parent(s) is going through a challenging time may find – on being taken to a child psychologist – that the search for evidence of attention deficit hyperactivity disorder involves the parent being asked to recall similar conduct. Evidence of past creativity or generosity will be ignored in a co-construction of a 'difficult' childhood to date.

Youthanasia

In the medieval period childhood in England formally ended at age 12. Fluctuations in meaning, however, are never new: 'In 1800 the meaning of childhood was ambiguous and not universally in demand. By 1914 the uncertainty had been virtually resolved and the identity largely determined, to the satisfaction of the middle class and the respectable working class ... each new construction ... may be observed in approximate chronological order as pertaining to Rousseauian Naturalism, Romanticism, Evangelicalism, the shift from wage-earning labour to "childhood", the reclamation of the juvenile delinquent, schooling ...'[9] Here, the perspective is limited; though class and respectability are parameters used by the author, race and religion are absent. For Jews or Hindus, rituals such as the bar mitzvah or arranged marriage are marks of the child becoming an adult, with no transitional period.

Parent–child relationships have been a focus of Psy since the late nineteenth century. Psycho-historian Lloyd deMause's 'periodisation' of modes of parent–child relations has been summarised as beginning with the infanticide mode (antiquity to fourth century AD), followed by the abandonment mode (fourth to thirteenth centuries AD), the ambivalent mode (fourteenth to seventeenth centuries), the intrusive mode (eighteenth century), the socialisation mode (nineteenth to mid-twentieth centuries) and finally the helping mode, starting in the mid-twentieth century and continuing.[10]

There is an element of myth-making to this reading. Certainly *some* ancient Greek and Roman parents would have killed their children, and children of slaves – as non-citizens – would have been easy targets. Similarly, numerous foundling hospitals were established in Europe during the 'abandonment' period, although no account is taken by deMause of the strenuous efforts of local village communities to provide as comfortable lives as possible for their charges, lives more secure than those possible in homes marked by the presence of too many siblings to feed.[11] The (admittedly truncated) summary of deMause's account also ignores dimensions of class, religion, race and gender.

However 'ambivalent' parents may have been during the medieval period, states and kingdoms seem to have recognised that children were, indeed, 'children' in the more contemporary sense. Myths concerning the so-called Children's Crusade, for example, have been shown to be false. Although people as young as 15 may have occasionally gone to war this was not common – peasant children were needed to farm the land and help their mothers if their fathers had gone to fight.[12] The fame of Joan of Arc (who led the relief of Orléans aged 17) and Edward the Black Prince (who at the age of 16 fought at the side of his father, Edward III, at the Battle of Crécy) spread because of their exceptional youth – it was unusual for adolescents to go into battle.

If child-soldiers were rare, child-workers were not. The extent of child labour in the industrialised north of England in the early nineteenth century has attained almost mythic status. Detailed by, amongst others, Friedrich Engels (himself a mill owner, albeit one who subsidised his friend and co-author Karl Marx), families lived in squalor with little to eat and children were to be found alongside their mothers in cotton mills. But the experience of agricultural workers was, arguably, just as severe. Under the 1840s' 'gang system' of labour in the eastern counties of England, children as young as four would walk up to eight miles to work in the fields from 8.30am to 5.30pm. They would return home to a small cottage, frequently with no flooring, to find an equally exhausted mother too tired (and poor) to prepare a meal.[13] At the same time, in the 'domestic industry' of knitting, embroidery, glove and button making children were earning a regular wage by age six. In contrast to the kind of child labour (eight-year-olds working up to 19 hours a day) that led to the first factory act of 1833, which theoretically prohibited employment of all those under nine, this domestic trade was invisible. Here, 'Hidden away ... thousands of children in rural areas worked factory hours every day.'[14]

There may have been marginal changes in education and employment law relating to children in Victorian England but for many children their lives were little altered. In 1885, for example, in order to prove that white slavery was a thriving industry, Stead of the *Pall Mall Gazette* was arrested for *buying* a 13-year-old girl in Marylebone, London.[15]

One history of childhood in the northern hemisphere might – for the sake of cohesion – be seen in terms of phases, wherein children were: 1) for millennia not much in evidence in any documentation unless the offspring of the rich (there is, for example, no birth certificate for William Shakespeare); 2) documented as cheap labour in the cotton, mining and domestic industries of the eighteenth and subsequent centuries (though the bones of child miners have even been found in the Neolithic Grimes' Graves in Norfolk); or 3) more recently, recorded as the victims of a combined 'war' against them with the Psy complex and arms industries as willing accomplices.

The twentieth and early twenty-first centuries might better deserve the sobriquet 'killing mode'. During the Armenian genocide in the second decade of the twentieth century, women, children and elderly people were removed from their homes and forced to march hundreds of miles without food or water to the desert of modern-day Syria.[16] Hundreds of thousands of people died on these forced marches and those who survived were put into concentration camps. Families were massacred indiscriminately.[17]

Analysis carried out for the research group Iraq Body Count found that 39 per cent of those killed in air raids by the US-led coalition were children. Of the fatalities caused by mortars, used by American and Iraqi government forces as well as insurgents, 42 per cent were children.[18] The 2009 report *The Weapons that Kill Civilians: Deaths of children and noncombatants in Iraq, 2003–2008* was compiled from a sample of 60,481 deaths in 14,196 events over a five-year period since the 2003 invasion. Civilian casualties from concentrated bouts of violence, such as the two sieges of Fallujah, were excluded.[19] In 2011 25 per cent of victims of landmines and explosive remnants of war were Iraqi children under the age of 14 years, and 23.9 per cent of the 80,000 casualties from failed cluster submunitions in 2007 were children under the age of 14.[20]

One outcome of the invasion of Iraq for school-age children is that Iraqi boys frequently now work to financially support the family instead of going to school. UNICEF estimates that one in nine children aged 5 to 14 years old work – polishing shoes, selling in the streets and pushing carriages.[21]

In Africa the 'childhoods' of many can be brutally short compared with those that might be considered 'typical' in the northern hemisphere. Since the start of the 'African War' in 1996, 5,400,000 have died in the Democratic Republic of Congo – 45,000 more die each month. The death toll is due to widespread disease and famine; half the individuals who have died are children under the age of five.[22]

These examples illustrate a few of the differences – historically and culturally – in what might be considered a 'normal' childhood, a period that for many is marked and frequently truncated by the actions of adults. The next section will look at how the Psy era of inscription and interiority has come to dominate the ways in which young persons are defined.

Psy and the 'normal' child

The Child Study Society formed in 1907 with the merging of the Child Study Association (founded in 1894) and the more medically/ statistically orientated Childhood Society (founded in 1896). The Child Study Society produced numerous reports on childhood, which was rapidly enveloped 'in a world of scientific experts of one sort or another'.[23] By the time of the onset of the First World War children were being involved 'in a consciously designed pursuit of the [British] national interest, which included … racial hygiene, responsible parenthood, social purity and preventive medicine'.[24] This type of control – via a language of individual responsibility and the construction of distinct selves with supposedly unique but quantifiable characteristics – has been called 'governmentality'. Governmentality is 'the ensemble formed by institutions, procedures, analyses and reflections, the calculations and tactics, that allow the exercise of this very specific albeit complex form of power, which has its target population'.[25]

A key facet of governmentality is the inscription of the self. The gaze of Psy has been fundamental to this inscription. Nikolas Rose suggests the origins of observational Psy praxis started with Darwin, James Sully (Grote Professor of the Philosophy of Mind and Logic at University College, London, and the person who called the founding meeting of the British Psychological Society in 1901), and Granville Stanley Hall, first president of the American Psychological Association.[26] All three observed and documented infants and drew parents into a disciplinary space in order to collate observations of their own children. Developmental psychology can be traced to the work of Arnold Gesell at Yale in 1911. By the 1920s Gesell's 'Psycho-clinic' had incorporated a small, well-lit laboratory sided by two-way mirrors. The experimenter and child could not see the observers and camera technician as the scientist (in white coat) was observed 'testing' the child.[27] Rose states, 'The child is here caught up within a complicated arrangement that will transform it into … [an] analysable object, within a particular rational scientific discourse (developmental psychology) making a particular kind of claim upon our attention – a claim to truth.'[28] Experiments of this type – work with patients, research on 'normal' subjects and more – has led to Psy inscribing a problematised self as disordered, abnormal or developmentally delayed.

A similar form of observation is maintained in the training of child psychologists, child analysts (who frequently observe parent–child interactions during training) and family therapists. For some critics this is Psy at its most naive: practitioners and experimenters act as if the experimental and observational context is irrelevant to the behaviour observed.

The widening expert gaze before the war set the context for the establishment of child guidance clinics in the 1920s and the emerging disciplines of child, educational and developmental psychology. All three were boosted by the advent of the Second World War and the opportunity to study the effects of evacuation from the major English cities of nearly one million unaccompanied children and half a million mothers with preschool children to non-industrial areas less likely to be bombed.

Foucault suggested that 'normality' is defined by a focus on the abnormal – a praxis that disguises the disciplinary nature of expert knowledge. Thus, child development 'milestones' or family 'stages' are identified by reference to failure to display the desired conduct. At its simplest this might be the notion that the 'average' family is a married couple with two children and that threats to this normative arrangement come from the increasing incidence of teenage pregnancy, gay marriage or single-parenthood. *Finding* this average family may prove difficult. Although the married-couple-plus-two-(point-four)-children has been with us in the UK since the 1950s, divorce statistics from that same decade reveal that this version of the nuclear family was not typical. In England and Wales in 1957, 23,785 marriages were dissolved or annulled. At the date of petition 7,995 were childless; another 1,567 had four or more children, 10 per cent of these when the wife was under 20 years old.[29]

A contemporary cross-cultural analysis reveals equally diverse norms for families and ages of parenthood. In comparisons of Europe, the US and Australasia rates of teenage motherhood vary widely. In 2012 Switzerland had the lowest birth rate with 3.4 births per 1,000 women aged 15–19 and Azerbaijan had the highest rate with 50 births. In 2012 the birth rate among young women was 16.1 per 1,000 women aged 15–19 in Australia, 24.9 in New Zealand and 29.4 in the United States.[30]

'Childcare' is frequently in the hands of those other than the biological parents. UK orphanages in the 1950s, for example, accepted refugees from the Hungarian uprising just as, today, foster carers are charged with (and assessed on) the care of neglected and abandoned children. Less dramatically, grandparents frequently care for their children's offspring to enable parents to earn an income. In New Zealand the fostering and adoption of children is a long-established Māori customary practice. Traditionally it was not uncommon for children to be tamaiti whāngai (reared by other members of the family), often by those who could not have children, or who wanted more children. Children were treated as the natural children of their whāngai parents and could inherit possessions and land. In some cases children were given to strengthen family ties. Children's connections to their natural parents were often maintained so they could move between families. In common with the majority of the world's population, Māori children can be promised as future husbands or wives for other children, a custom known as taumau or tomo. A betrothed girl is known as a puhi and carefully watched over during her adolescence.[31]

One technique of family Psy experts is to use patients (*pace* Foucault) in order to illustrate stages in child or family development. Thus, a chapter on 'The family life cycle' in one 1980s guide to 'normal family processes' suggests that – in middle-class America in the late twentieth century – families move from stage 1 (the unattached young adult) to stage 6 (the family in later life). According to the authors, 'acceptance', 'adjustment' and 're-alignment of relationships' are necessary at each transitional stage. They go on to illustrate failures in these processes by reference to four case vignettes.[32]

This reading of (failed) 'normality' by use of clinical material is so common in Psy literature that some Psy professionals may have lost touch with the fact that these kinds of data can tell us nothing about either normality *or* so-called average families and development. From Anna Freud to Alice Miller, via John Bowlby, Donald Winnicott and Bruno Bettelheim, theories of children's lives and experience have depended on particular views on interiority already held by the expert.[33] Neither Freud nor Winnicott had children. The latter's 25-year marriage to his wife Alice was unconsummated.[34] He had been trained by Melanie Klein, whose estrangement from her daughter Melitta Schmideberg was so complete that the latter ignored her mother's funeral, preferring instead to deliver a lecture elsewhere, 'wearing flamboyant red boots'.[35] Bettelheim was estranged from one of his daughters before he committed suicide in 1990 aged 86. Since his death he has been accused by ex-patients of the University of Chicago's Sonia Shankman Orthogenic School of physically abusing them.

Evidence that Bettelheim and others were all too human in their position as inspirational theorists and unpleasant or flawed individuals is not evidence that their theories were wrong. The difficulty here is that there can *be* no evidence of generally applicable theories of human development. Notions of interiority and individuality join with concepts such as personality to make the child a tabula rasa for theoreticians committed to untestable notions such as 'development' ('change' would be more accurate) or invisible entities such as 'the id' or 'the superego'.

The (contextual) uncritical acceptance of gendered societal roles by, amongst others, Freud, Erik Erikson and Bettelheim has been noted by various critics. In addition:

> The first reason for psychology's failure to understand what people are and how they act is that psychology has looked for inner traits when it should have been looking for social context; the second reason for psychology's failure is that the theoreticians of personality have generally been clinicians and psychiatrists, and they have never considered it necessary to have evidence in support of their theories.[36]

I suspect for the majority of parents the first port of call for help with children – from babysitting to bed-wetting – is relatives, other parents or friends. The psychologist and author Dorothy Rowe has given me some invaluable advice. Some of her books even feature my children.[37] We were confused and concerned about the point at which my first daughter should be toilet trained, and Dorothy suggested, 'She'll let you know when she's ready.' Later, when my daughter was asking to be allowed to sleep with her mum and dad – usually between us – Dorothy advised, 'Remember, everything in childhood is a phase.' It is an aphorism that could describe any point in someone's life, but one which relieved the worry at the time. It is also something parents of children showing signs of unwanted conduct might bear in mind. Too often the conduct leads to a search for expert opinion, entry into the Psy system, diagnosis and a career as a patient. Allowing change at the child's pace can be too challenging for some parents whose expectancies of the 'right' age to sleep through the night or stop wetting the bed are as constrained as the right age for a child's bar or bat mitzvah.

The next section discusses some of the potential ensuing consequences when concerned parents ask Psy experts for assistance.

From inscription to prescription

A scientific discourse demands that any diagnosis be reliable; that is, observers must agree on what they observe and agree on the diagnosis, an agreement known as inter-rater reliability. The first three editions of the *Diagnostic and Statistical Manual of Mental Disorders* (*DSM*) categorised conduct under diagnostic headings with very low inter-rater reliability. One might conjecture that for a supposed scientific endeavour this was embarrassing. The solution for the American Psychiatric Association was to remove all reference to inter-rater reliability for subsequent editions. Diagnostic praxis should also be valid – the extent to which diagnosis predicts behaviour. Citing numerous authors, David Stein suggests that diagnoses have *no* predictive, internal, external or concurrent validity. They are 'about as accurate as a Ouija Board'.[38] Construct validity is, by necessity, impossible within Psy. Like 'connectedness' or 'love', Psy constructs such as personality or the unconscious are not available to physical investigation and, as hypothetical notions, have no construct validity. You can neither hurry love, nor touch it.

These concerns are emphasised in only a minority of educative programmes for Psy students. In the US, for example, diagnoses and Psy interventions are supported by psychometric testing, and the majority of accredited psychology doctoral programmes continue to teach 'assessment'. This involves learning to administer projective tests such as the Rorschach or personality tests such as the Minnesota Multiphasic Personality Inventory (MMPI) and Thematic Apperception Test (TAT) which has a version for children. At best the Rorschach and TAT can reliably predict behaviour less than 10 per cent of the time.[39]

It has been argued elsewhere that the use of diagnosis and psychometric testing owes more to the demands of research communities and publishers than any commitment to science. 'Science' is, for the majority, a trope bringing cultural capital and the illusion of expert authority to the user.[40]

Lloyd deMause's twentieth-century 'helping mode' might be entitled the 'inscription and interference mode'. Emil Kraepelin used the term 'manic depressive psychosis' – the first of his formal diagnostic categories and the forerunner of bipolar disorder – in 1896. The conduct involved cycles of intense mania (grandiosity, irritability, etc.) and depression (oversleeping, suicidality, etc.). As with any Psy inscription these descriptors were wholly subjective and based on reports from relatives, physicians and, sometimes, the inscribed patient. This last was problematic as one supposed aspect of 'psychosis' was a lack of insight. Since the mid-twentieth century those so inscribed have been administered a toxic salt – lithium carbonate. Unsurprisingly, lithium has a calming effect on a condition regarded as a genetically induced brain disorder. There is, however, no reliable evidence of either a genetic factor or brain dysfunction – until the patient has started to take the medication – in the majority of Psy diagnoses which are, in any case, metaphorical constructs.

For the World Health Organization, using the International Classification (ICD-11), bipolar disorder is seen as rare. In the US the preferred classification system, which for insurance payment purposes uses the same codes as ICD, is the *Diagnostic and Statistical Manual (DSM)*. Since the broadening of the criteria for a diagnosis of bipolar disorder in 2000 with the introduction of *DSM-IV-TR*, diagnosis of the disorder in the US has 'soared'.[41]

The worldwide prevalence estimates of attention deficit hyperactivity disorder (ADHD)/hyperkinetic disorder (HD) are highly heterogeneous. Authors of a 2007 global prevalence study searched MEDLINE and PsycINFO databases from January 1978 to December 2005 and reviewed textbooks and reference lists of the studies selected. They contacted authors of relevant articles from North America, South America, Europe, Africa, Asia, Oceania, and the Middle East. The literature search generated 9,105 records, and 303 full-text articles were reviewed. Included were 102 studies comprising 171,756 subjects from all world regions; the ADHD/HD worldwide-pooled prevalence was 5.29 per cent. This estimate was associated with significant variability. Geographic location was associated with significant variability between estimates from North America and both Africa and the Middle East. No significant differences were found between Europe and North America.[42]

In the US from 2000 to 2010, the number of physician outpatient visits in which ADHD was diagnosed increased 66 per cent from 6.2 million to 10.4 million visits. Psycho-stimulants have remained the dominant treatment, used in 96 per cent of treatment visits in 2000 and 87 per cent of treatment visits in 2010. During the decade, the management of ADHD shifted away from paediatricians and towards psychiatrists (from 24% to 36% of all visits).[43]

Twenty years ago two child psychology research groups in the US claimed that many children diagnosed with ADHD should be regarded as bipolar. One result of this claim is that children exhibiting 'stormy episodes of "mania" lasting only minutes' can be diagnosed with bipolar disorder. Despite reservations concerning the wholly theoretical link to adult bipolar disorder the American Association of Child and Adolescent Psychiatry's (AACAP) *Practice Parameters* recommend major tranquillisers and anticonvulsants as the first line treatment, in part to prevent the disorder continuing into adulthood.[44] The disorder is marketed through Facebook pages, websites and literature for professionals, parents and children. Two authors of the AACAP document disclose ties to the pharmaceutical industry. One, Robert Findling, has links with 16 drug manufacturers including AstraZeneca, GlaxoSmithKline and Lilly.[45] The doyen and, some would say, instigator of the rise in diagnosis, is the leader of the Harvard Research Group, Joseph Biederman. It has been suggested that drug industry payments to his group 'can only be presumed to run into the millions'.[46]

Elizabeth Roberts, a psychiatrist, describes paediatric bipolar disorder as the latest 'diagnosis du jour', remarking that the rise in diagnosis rates has been 'meteoric'. Noting that major tranquillisers (in her terms, 'antipsychotic' medication) are frequently prescribed for children with the diagnosis, she comments that there was a fivefold increase in prescriptions over the period 1995 to 2002.[47] Her response to the diagnostic project has not been to discard diagnoses. In offering a case example of a child (six-year-old 'Andy') *diagnosed* with ADHD and referred by a *teacher* to a paediatrician who prescribed Ritalin, Roberts instead inscribes the boy as 'having reactive attachment disorder' and prescribes antidepressants.[48]

As with ADHD (and, now adult ADD), the criteria for inscribing autism – first described by Leo Kanner, the 'father of child psychiatry', in 1943 – continue to change, drawing more children into the Psy embrace. The October 2014 issue of *The Psychologist* was devoted exclusively to 'Autism: Myth and reality'.[49] An introductory article by Uta Frith suggests that autism is a 'puzzle' solvable by considering 'myths and realities'. She goes on to say, 'we now know that autism can occur at all levels of intellectual ability, including very superior levels.'[50] The author cites 'profound social communication problems' as the 'core of autism'.[51] Noting that Asperger syndrome no longer appears in the *DSM*, Frith suggests that the expansion of criteria for inclusion in the grouping autism spectrum disorder (ASD) means that some people with 'problems in social relationships and other features reminiscent of autism' have been labelled Asperger's but 'actually belong to a different category', which remains 'sadly' ill-defined and 'even part of neurotypical individual variation'.[52] Frith continues, 'Many psychologists and psychiatrists had only just become aware of autism, and now they had to embrace a whole autistic spectrum.' The lack of validity of the concept does not deter Frith from then remarking, 'The impact is still felt even if the label Asperger syndrome no longer appears in the 5th edition of the *Diagnostic and Statistical Manual* of the American Psychiatric Association.'[53] The nature of the 'impact' is not explored in detail, though, like autism and autistic spectrum disorder, Asperger syndrome has entered the vernacular. A lack of validity is not a bar to such terms entering ordinary discourse. Boyle has demonstrated that it is the *repetition* of technical language (for example, the everyday use of terms such as schizophrenia or 'clinical' depression in the mass media) that gives words in the Psy lexis the appearance of referring to real disease or disorder *without the need* to establish on scientific grounds their existence.[54] Frith's two-page article uses the word autism *33* times.

The article maintains tropes of science, expertise and allusions to mind or brain for an audience dominated by similar vested interest and conversant with the same tropes. Similar rhetorical devices appear in Patricia Howlin's later article on understanding autism after 70 years of research.[55] She notes the origins of 'the condition', going on to remark that subsequent to the inclusion of 'the disorder' in the *DSM-III* of 1980, prevalence has steadily risen – from 0.4 per 1,000 to 14.7 per 1,000. Addressing perceived fears of 'an epidemic of autism' as mythic, Howlin claims that the increased incidence reflects increased professional and public 'awareness'. Perhaps again attempting to diffuse alarm she notes Rutter's work demonstrating the 'differences between autism and schizophrenia'.[56] This raises one straw man against another – a classic rhetorical move – as neither schizophrenia nor autism are valid entities it is *only* possible to suggest they are similar to or different from each other via definition. Changing the definition of the terms will exclude some individuals and include others; no 'research' is necessary. The process is evident, for example, in the ever-changing number of people living below the 'poverty line' – a concept invented by Charles Booth in 1886 and manipulated at will by British governments ever since.

Howlin acknowledges: 'There are currently no imaging techniques that can reliably identify autism at an individual level.' Theories of 'causation' – parental 'pathology', organic conditions and genetics – are shown to be either unproven or common across other diagnostic clusters. 'Treatments' show equal variability and lack of impact whether based on psychoanalytic or behavioural theories. Unsurprisingly, a 20-hour-*per-week* two-*year* treatment programme focusing on communication problems 'suggests' improvement in some modalities if measured against 'un-treated' children. Acknowledging that there is 'great variation in treatment response', Howlin says that generalisation of treatment effects to new skills is 'limited' and there is 'no evidence of long term impact'. Despite this, Howlin suggests a broadening of the target treatment population to include less affluent families. The gaze is thus extended *from* the middle classes *to* the working or unemployed classes *in the absence* of the gaze having positive results for the population observed. This is consistent with Foucault's original conception of the gaze offering the more powerful professional and middle classes a further tool in disciplining the less powerful poor. In acting as the disciplinary corpus, professionals are themselves disciplined via an insistence on particular language and membership of professional bodies.

In summary, identification and treatment of the so-called disorder has been haphazard and unsuccessful for 70 years. In order to retain the gaze, not only are the characteristics of autism to be widened (*pace*

Frith) but so too are the age and class parameters. A more *scientific* approach might be to conclude that Psy has no place in interfering with the lives of children (and adults) who are struggling in ways increasingly described as 'autistic'. Howlin uses a simple rhetorical device to draw an opposing conclusion, stating, '*If* the advances in comprehensive treatment programmes for very young children can be applied across the lifespan, then the current generation of children with autism *may* face a more positive future' (my italics).[57] It is a statement of hope over experience and cannot be justified in her own – scientific – terms.

An inscription of autism can, for many children, lead to the prescription of psychiatric drugs, frequently major tranquillisers. Such prescription is regarded as an appropriate first response to unwanted behaviour. In the US almost eight-and-a-half million children up to 17 years old are now on psychiatric drugs having been inscribed with ADHD, anxiety, bipolar, depression, or other diagnoses such as oppositional defiant disorder (ODD). Over one million are infants, toddlers, pre-schoolers and kindergartners; 274,804 are one year old or less, 370,778 are aged two to three, and 500,948 are four to five years old.[58]

Children in industrialised countries are part of a Psy industry that trades in their distress or disturbing conduct and sometimes in the children themselves – for example, when a private social care company bids successfully for a child care contract involving institutionalised children. Marketing of Psy services for children uses tropes of 'health', 'disorder', or 'wellbeing' in order to attract customers and patients. Services are bound within a linguistic discourse of interiority and inscription that makes inevitable the use of the health/ill health lexicon.

The Child Psychotherapy Trust, for example, was set up in 1987 to promote child psychotherapy services in the UK National Health Service. Although it ceased to operate in 2004 some of its leaflets are still available from an NHS website. One includes the following statement: 'When the child's behaviour is affected most or all of the time, there may be a serious problem … more difficult to tackle than most … attention deficit disorder (ADD) or attention deficit hyperactivity disorder (ADHD).' It continues, 'Only in the most severe cases will drug treatments be required.' It then encourages the parent to 'please contact your GP or health visitor or local child guidance or child and family clinic.'[59]

Private Psy services for children and families are also readily available. The Institute for Neuro-Physiological Psychology (INPP), for example, is based in Chester, UK. It was founded 'with the aim of researching into the effect of immaturity in the functioning of the central nervous system on specific learning difficulties and adults suffering from agoraphobia and panic disorder'. The INPP website suggests that 'neuro-developmental delay' (NDD) can be 'an underlying factor' in many cases where children have been described as having a learning disability or diagnosed with ADHD. The site offers a 'free NDD child screening test'.[60]

As noted above, the inscription of children via diagnosis is ubiquitous. The Psy industries depend on a discourse of interiority and disorder which – for all its apparent scientific roots – is dependent on the judgement of Psy professionals. That judgement is not reliable and, even when supported by the techno-armoury of psychologists, is not valid. The discourse has penetrated the public lexicon, and teachers and parents join with journalists in their use of Psy terminology. The context for professionals no less than children is thus one of inscription and prescription. Individual professionals can add to their cultural capital by embracing that discourse.

Western Australia, for example, has had a prescribed stimulants monitoring system in place for over a decade. When the system was first introduced it revealed that one single paediatrician prescribed to 2,077 children in 17 months from August 2003 to December 2004. This paediatrician was 'encouraged' to retire from prescribing and his subsequent retirement was immediately followed by a significant decrease in child prescribing rates. The overall reduction in stimulant prescribing to children in Western Australia had until recently shown a sharp fall. In 2011, however, *one* clinician (a psychiatrist) was responsible for prescribing to 1,473 patients (1,346 adults and 127 children), causing a 'spike' in the figures.[61]

Psychoactive drugs are only part of the story in relation to Psy's involvement with children. There are some 600 psychotherapies.[62] Children can be subjected to the majority of psychotherapeutics and, within the family, can receive a wide variety of family and systems counselling. Children may receive counselling via schools after events such as a school coach crash or a school shooting, or where sexual abuse has been identified. The praxis has been extensively critiqued in relation to untestable theorising, abuse by therapists and outcome. In the Fort Bragg Demonstration Project, inpatient and outpatient psychological services were offered to over 42,000 children and adolescents for five years. Patients were assessed via self-report (most were satisfied with their treatment) and psychometric assessment during and after treatment.

A reader in the professional camp might perhaps defensively turn the accusation of scientism against the research in its reliance on psychometric data. Nonetheless, the study has been heralded as an example of one of the few research projects of its type to use a sufficiently large sample; a qualitative methodology would have proved immensely costly (as it is, the study cost $80 million[63]). Tana Dineen cites the downbeat conclusions of the Fort Bragg project's authors that 'the assumption that clinical services are in any way effective might be erroneous', and, 'although substantial evidence for the efficacy of psychotherapy under laboratory-like conditions exists, there is scant evidence of its effectiveness in real-life community settings (i.e. outside of the research setting)'.[64]

The rights of children

Some Psy professionals take up a rights discourse in an effort to reduce the impact of Psy praxis. Clinical psychologist and psychiatrist allies of organisations such as the World Network for Users and Survivors of Psychiatry promote the position of psychiatric survivors as citizens. Similarly, clinical psychology has been represented amongst feminist critics and those concerned with the rights of young people coerced into arranged marriage or victims of torture.[65]

'Children have the right to live' is Article 6 of the UN Convention on the Rights of the Child. All UN member states except for the United States have ratified the Convention (Somalia is in the process of finalising ratification of the Convention). In the UK the relevant act came into force in January 1992. There are 54 articles detailing the rights and expectations on governments, professionals and families to uphold the rights of those under the age of 18. In the UK, for the purposes of the convention, the cut-off from childhood to adulthood is taken to be 17. Article 1 states that states should be encouraged 'to review the age of majority if it is set below 18 and to increase the level of protection for all children under 18'. In the UK any such moves to date have been invisible to the public.[66]

The convention legitimises involvement by the UN where there are clear breaches of the convention. The implied governmentality by parents and government bodies is a more insidious process. Documents of this type can be relatively easy to read, while making recommendations that are difficult to follow. Article 16, for example, gives those under 18 the 'Right to privacy'. From children living in crowded homes to journalists writing personal stories about their own children this right is ignored. Article 3 demands that, 'All adults should do what is best for children.' This opens up a parenting Pandora's box where experts and parents can debate the benefits of anything from homework to smacking.

Article 5 (Parental guidance) prompts governments to 'respect the rights and responsibilities of families to direct and guide their children so that, as they grow, they learn to use their rights properly', while not 'pushing them [children] to make choices with consequences that they are too young to handle'. Under Article 29 signatories agree 'that the education of the child shall be directed to: (a) The development of the child's personality, talents and mental and physical abilities to their fullest potential … (c) The development of respect … for the national values of the country in which the child is living, the country from which he or she may originate, and for civilizations different from his or her own … and (e) The development of respect for the natural environment'.[67] These are tall orders and arose in a context where in some countries *survival* of children was an issue. The trope of 'development' and interiorised notion of 'personality' appear, now aligned with impossible-to-define notions of 'national values' and potentially contradictory appeals to 'respect'. Trees may need to be torn down to build safer housing for some children.

The United Kingdom government made its first report to the Committee on the Rights of the Child in January 1995. Concerns raised by the committee included the growth in child poverty and inequality, the extent of violence towards children, the use of custody for young offenders, the low age of criminal responsibility, and the lack of opportunities for children and young people to express views. The 2002 report of the committee expressed similar concerns, including the welfare of children in custody, unequal treatment of asylum seekers and the negative impact of poverty on children's rights. In September 2008 the UK government withdrew its reservations and agreed to the convention in these respects.

The 2002 report's criticism of the legal defence of 'reasonable chastisement' of children by parents, which the committee described as 'a serious violation of the dignity of the child', was rejected by the UK government. The Minister for Children, Young People and Families commented that while fewer parents are using smacking as a form of discipline, the majority said they would not support a ban.[68] How the minister knew the position of the majority in relation to smacking is not recorded.

Diagnosis and inscription are used interchangeably in this chapter though children are inscribed using tropes such as 'innocent' as well as formal diagnostic terms. Inscription is the preferred description of the naming process as it implies a more visceral act; like inscribing on tombstones, these inscriptions will outlive the child. Inscribed within case notes, children obtain new identities of 'other', disabled or damaged. This re-identification is equally lasting and, coincidentally, does not comply with Article 8 of the Convention on the Rights of the Child.

The Convention also states that children have the right to have their views taken into account on all matters that affect them. In the UK, user and carer involvement in all aspects of service design and delivery is supposedly a central feature of the modernisation agenda for the NHS. These principles were echoed in the National Service Frameworks (NSFs) for mental health[69] and for children, young people and maternity services.[70] The latter was published in 2004 and a ten-year review planned.

The guidance includes prompts to involve children in the mental health services they use. It has been suggested that the term 'service user' is a political tool designed to disguise the power imbalance between psychology and recipients – when a CAMHS (child and adolescent mental health service) implements user involvement, it is most commonly in the form of service evaluation.[71] Parents have tended to be used as spokespeople for their children in these studies. In addition, research has shown that parents' assessments of their children's wellbeing and opinions are frequently inaccurate.[72] Children have been involved in developing information leaflets[73] and the recruitment of staff.[74] The re-inscription of children as service consultants – though not 'appointing officers' – here places people too young to vote in the position of co-selecting adult government employees.

By contrast, the non-profit organisation Imagine Chicago began in September 1992 with a design team consisting of educators, corporate and media executives, philanthropists, community organisers, youth developers, economists, religious leaders, and social service providers, under the direction of Bliss Browne, a mother of three, Episcopal priest and former Division Head of the First National Bank of Chicago. Their aim, via 'appreciative' enquiry with distantiated youth and gang leaders in one of the most violent and rundown areas of the city, was to create an environment that might enable young people to thrive rather than go on to a life of crime and incarceration. Over 20 years later many of the goals have been achieved and the project has expanded to embrace similar enterprises in other cities.[75]

Think about the children

If childhood is a myth, children are not. They live in a world dominated by adults, the vast majority of whom are the servants of power.[76] Psychiatric assault via medication and electrocution of young people continues unabated.[77] Inscription of children by Psy professionals has now been generalised within a public discourse whereby children are no longer excited but 'manic', no longer sad but 'depressed'. The media focuses on interiority in its use of terms such as 'evil' or 'innocent' when children are involved in crime or are hurt by others. Children continue to be victims of war and, in some countries, are soldiers or bombers. Slavery or sexual assault – frequently re-inscribed as 'abuse' – are as common now as in the nineteenth century. The distantiation of children to 'care homes' has done little to protect them from assault. In the early 1990s I was involved in an investigation and eventual closure of a 'care home' in Shropshire for orphaned and unwanted children. Referred by social workers across the border in Wales, children were subjected to humiliation *as part of the programme* and there were several incidents of assault and suicide. The building has since been converted into highly desirable apartments. During the last decade of the twentieth century 150 cases of sexual and physical assault were proven in 18 Welsh children's homes between 1963 and 1992. In the US children have killed other children and adults in widely publicised school shootings, and in Asia children continue to work in conditions of low pay reminiscent of the mine workers in the Rand in South Africa at the turn of the nineteenth and twentieth centuries.[78]

'Childhood' remains mythic – a time when the adult-dominated world can harm, hinder or help in the name of 'good' parenting or 'evidence-based' interventions. No qualifications are required to become a parent and the qualification of *being* a parent is not required of Psy professionals. As I have discussed elsewhere, a Psy professional who is also a parent works in a context where parenthood is, in any case, no guarantee that Psy interventions will be beneficent, and the perpetual 'othering' via inscription of child patients creates a distance (described as 'professional boundaries') whereby the professional is less likely to respond as a person touched by the child's plight.[79]

In wealthier countries children and parents are besieged by advice columns, blogs and TV programmes suggesting the desirability of 'quality time' with each other, the necessity to succeed educationally and the importance of achieving 'developmental' milestones. Any failure may result in appeals to *more* expert advice and intervention.

My intention is this chapter has been to outline some of the myth-making around continually redefined notions of childhood and to summarise some of the consequences for children of those redefinitions. One historical-cultural reading suggests that the lives of children are no safer or protected than a few centuries ago although, as noted above, the nature of ordinary life for children prior to 1800 is difficult to ascertain due to a lack of source materials. A child born in the Democratic Republic of Congo has a 50 per cent chance of living to the age of five. One born in the US may have shot someone by age six and a child of similar age in the UK may have been referred by a primary school teacher for a prospective Psy diagnosis. These incidents from the lives of children *are* far more common than a century ago. Childhood cannot be realistically described as an age of innocence.

In Rousseauian Romantic vein an appeal could be made to adults to be more aware of the impact of our actions on children. As Richie Havens put it: 'We say we love, we say we care, we say we know ... think about the children.'[80] Such an appeal would take its place alongside many similar appeals from politicians to children's charities. And, it does rather assume that adults care.

Endnotes

1. Szasz, T. (1994). Cruel Compassion: Psychiatric control of society's unwanted. Chichester: John Wiley & Sons.
2. The London 2012 Paralympics privileged a particular version of the disability identity where young people were consistently hailed as 'courageous' in their pursuit of athletic excellence. For potential Paralympic competitors, being marked as *more* disabled is, due to the compensatory points system, a much sought-after advantage to the young athletes. See: Burns, J. (2013). *Won't Get Fooled Again: Psychology and the Paralympics* [conference paper]. Presented at I Can See for Miles: The future of Psy, a celebratory conference in memory of Professor Mark Rapley. University of East London, 13 April 2013.
3. Boyle, D. (2000). *The Tyranny of Numbers: Why counting can't make us happy.* London: Harper Collins.
4. Philippe Aries argues that childhood itself is a concept common to all social classes in the northern hemisphere only since the early twentieth century. For Aries childhood is an 'invention'. See Calder, J. (2005). Histories of Child Abuse. In C. Newnes & N. Radcliffe (Eds) *Making and Breaking Children's Lives* (pp. 15–29). Ross-on-Wye: PCCS Books.
5. Kitzinger, J. (1997). Who are you kidding? Children, power and the struggle against sexual abuse. In A. James & A. Prout (Eds) *Constructing and Reconstructing Childhood: Contemporary issues in the sociological study of childhood* (pp. 165–189). London: Routledge Falmer, p. 167
6. BBC News from Elsewhere (2015). Russia: Child classics removed from library. Available at http://www.bbc.co.uk/news/blogs-news-from-elsewhere-32070271 (retrieved 21 March 2015).

7. Healy, D. & Le Noury, J. (2007). Bipolar disorder by proxy? The case of pediatric bipolar disorder. In S. Olfman (Ed.) *Bipolar Children: Cutting-edge controversy, insights and research* (pp. 12–27). Oxford: Praeger.
8. Leighton, H. R. (1910). *Memorials of Old Durham.* London: George Allen. Quoted in Roud, S. (2003). *The Penguin Guide to the Superstitions of Britain and Ireland.* Harmondsworth: Penguin Books, p. 436.
9. Hendrick, H. (1997). Constructions and reconstructions of British childhood: An interpretative study, 1900 to the present. In James & Prout op. cit. pp. 33–60, p. 35.
10. Calder, J. (2005). Histories of child abuse. In C. Newnes and N. Radcliffe (Eds) *Making and Breaking Children's Lives* (pp. 15–23). Ross-on-Wye: PCCS Books, p. 22.
11. See Goldberg, A. (1999). *Sex, Religion and the Making of Modern Madness: The Eberbach asylum and German society, 1815–1849.* New York: Oxford University Press.
12. Alvarez, S. (2014). Teenagers at war during the Middle Ages. Available at http://deremilitari.org/2014/03/teenagers-at-war-during-the-middle-ages/ (retrieved 19 March 2015).
13. Fletcher, R. (1962). *Britain in the Sixties: The family and marriage.* Harmondsworth: Penguin.
14. Pinchbeck, I. (1930). *Women Workers and the Industrial Revolution 1750–1850.* London: Routledge & Kegan Paul. Quoted in Fletcher, 1962, ibid. p. 85.
15. Boyle, D. (2000). *The Tyranny of Numbers: Why counting can't make us happy.* London: Harper Collins.
16. United Human Right Council (n.d.). Armenian Genocide. Available at http://www.unitedhumanrights.org/genocide/armenian_genocide.htm (retrieved 13 July 2013); Adalian, R. P. (n.d.). Armenian genocide. Armenian National Institute. Available at http://www.armenian-genocide.org/genocide.html (retrieved 18 July 2013).
17. Beecroft, R. H. (2013). Armenian genocide. Available at http://worldwithoutgenocide.org/genocides-and-conflicts/armenian-genocide (retrieved 15 March 2015).
18. Sengupta, K. (2009). Iraq air raids hit mostly women and children. Available at http://www.independent.co.uk/news/world/middle-east/iraq-air-raids-hit-mostly-women-and-children-1669282.html (retrieved 15 March 2015).
19. Kentane, B., (2012). The children of Iraq: Was the price worth it? Available at http://www.globalresearch.ca/the-children-of-iraq-was-the-price-worth-it/30760 (retrieved 15 March 2015).
20. Moving ahead to improve lives of Iraqis affected by landmines (2011). Available at http://www.uniraq.org/newsroom/getarticle.asp?ArticleID=1495 (retrieved 16 March 2015).
21. Fallen off the agenda? More and better aid needed for Iraq recovery (2010). Available at http://www.internal-displacement.org/assets/library/Middle-East/Iraq/pdf/Iraq-more-and-better-aid-needed-jul-2010.pdf (retrieved 16 March 2015).
22. World Without Genocide (n.d.). Democratic Republic of the Congo. Available at http://worldwithoutgenocide.org/genocides-and-conflicts/congo (retrieved 16 March 2015).
23. Hendrick, 1997, p. 49. See note 9.
24. Ibid.
25. Foucault, M. (1979). On governmentality. *Ideology and Consciousness, 6,* 5–22, p. 20.
26. Rose, N. (1989). *Governing the Soul: The shaping of the private self.* London: Routledge.
27. Ibid. See Plate 1, p. 143.
28. Ibid. p. 144.
29. Extracted from Registrar General of England and Wales (1957). *Registrar General's Statistical Review of England and Wales, 1957: Part II: Tables, Civil.* London: HMSO. Table 34, p. 54.

30. Office for National Statistics (2012). International comparisons of teenage births. Available at http://www.ons.gov.uk/ons/rel/vsob1/births-by-area-of-usual-residence-of-mother--england-and-wales/2012/sty-international-comparisons-of-teenage-pregnancy.html (retrieved 18 March 2015).
31. Higgins, R. & Meredith, P. (2014). Ngā tamariki: Māori childhoods: Maori children's upbringing. In *Te Ara: The Encyclopedia of New Zealand*. Available at htp://www.teara.govt.nz/en/nga-tamariki-maori-childhoods/page-2 (retrieved 18 March 2015).
32. McGoldrick, M. & Carter, E. A. (1982). The family life cycle. In F. Walsh (Ed.) *Normal Family Processes* (pp. 167–195). New York: Guilford Press, p. 176.
33. Rose, 1989. See note 26.
34. Kahr, B. (1995). Ethical dilemmas of the psycho-analytical biographer: The case of Donald Winnicott. Available at http://www.human-nature.com/free-associations/kahr.html (retrieved 23 March 2015).
35. Grosskurth, P. (1986). *Melanie Klein: Her world and her work.* Cambridge, MA: Harvard University Press, p. 461.
36. Weisstein, N. (1968). Psychology constructs the Female. Available at http://www.uic.edu/orgs/cwluherstory/CWLUArchive/psych.html (retrieved 25 October 2013).
37. Rowe, D. (2007). *My Dearest Enemy, My Dangerous Friend: Making and breaking sibling bonds.* London: Routledge.
38. Stein, D. (2012). *The Psychology Industry Under the Microscope!* Plymouth, UK: University Press of America Inc., p. 48.
39. Ibid. p. 7.
40. Newnes, C. (2015). *Inscription, Diagnosis and Deception in the Mental Health Industry: How Psy governs us all.* Basingstoke: Palgrave Macmillan.
41. Olfman, S. (2007). Bipolar children: Cutting-edge controversy. In S. Olfman (Ed.) *Bipolar Children: Cutting-edge controversy, insights and research* (pp. 1–11). Oxford: Praeger.
42. Polanczyk, G., Silva de Lima, M., Lessa Horta, D. B., Biederman, J. & Rohde, L. A. (2007). The worldwide prevalence of ADHD: A systematic review and metaregression analysis. *The American Journal of Psychiatry, 164* (6) 942–948.
43. Garfield, C. F., Dorsey, E. R., Zhu, S., Huskamp, H. A., Conti, R., Dusetzina, S. B., Higashi, A., Perrin, J. M., Kornfield, R. & Alexander, G. C. (2012). Trends in attention deficit hyperactivity disorder ambulatory diagnosis and medical treatment in the United States, 2000–2010. *Academic Pediatrics, 12* (2) 110–116.
44. Healy & Le Noury, 2007, p. 7. See note 7.
45. Ibid.
46. Diller, P. (2007). But don't call it science. In S. Olfman (Ed.) *Bipolar Children: Cutting-edge controversy, insights and research* (pp. 28–45). Oxford: Praeger.
47. Roberts, E. (2007). The childhood bipolar epidemic: Brat or bipolar? In S. Olfman (Ed.) *Bipolar Children: Cutting-edge controversy, insights and research* (pp. 64–82). Oxford: Praeger, p. 65.
48. Ibid. p. 73.
49. British Psychological Society (2014). Autism: Myth and reality. *The Psychologist, 27* (10) 718–800.
50. Frith, U. (2014). Autism: Are we any closer to explaining the enigma? *The Psychologist, 27* (10) 744–745.
51. Ibid. p. 744.
52. Ibid.
53. Ibid.
54. Boyle, M. (2008). Can we bear to live without the medical model? Paper presented at

De-Medicalising Misery II conference on 16 December 2008, University College London.
55. Howlin, P. (2014). A continuing journey. *The Psychologist, 27* (10) 796–798.
56. Rutter, M. (1968). Concepts of autism: A review of research. *Journal of Child Psychology and Psychiatry, 9* (1) 1–25.
57. Howlin, 2014, p. 797. See note 55.
58. Corrigan, M. W. (2015). Mind-bottling malarkey, medicine or malpractice? Available at https://www.psychologytoday.com/blog/kids-being-kids/201503/mind-bottling-malarkey-medicine-or-malpractice (retrieved 15 March 2015).
59. Understanding your overactive child (n.d.). Available at http://www.understandingchildhood.net/posts/understanding-your-overactive-child/ (retrieved 12 March 2015).
60. INPP (n.d.). Attention deficit disorder (ADD). Available at http://www.inpp.org.uk/intervention-adults-children/help-by-diagnosis/attention-deficit-disorder/ (retrieved 15 March 2015).
61. Whitely, M. (2012). Speed up and sit still. Available at http://www.speedupsitstill.com/spike-western-australian-adhd-child-prescribing-defies-long-term-trend-2 (retrieved 1 April 2015).
62. Feltham, C. (2013). *Counselling and Counselling Psychology: A critical examination.* Ross-on-Wye: PCCS Books.
63. Bickman, L. (1996). A continuum of care: More is not always better. *American Psychologist, 51* (7) 689–701.
64. Bickman, L., Summerfelt, W. T., Firth, J. & Douglas, S. (1997). The Stark County Evaluation Project: Baseline results of a randomized experiment. In D. Northrup & C. Nixon (Eds) *Evaluating Mental Health Services: How do programs for children 'work' in the real world?* (pp. 231–259). Newbury Park, CA: Sage Publications. Quoted in Dineen, T. (1999). *Manufacturing Victims: What the psychology industry is doing to people.* London: Constable, p. 128.
65. See, for example, Patel, N. (2011). Justice and reparation for torture survivors. *The Journal of Critical Psychology, Counselling and Psychotherapy, 11* (3) 132–145; and Stenfert Kroese, B. & Taylor, F. (2011). 'It's OK, you get used to it': Forced marriage and learning disabilities. *The Journal of Critical Psychology, Counselling and Psychotherapy, 11* (3) 154–162.
66. United Nations Human Rights (1990). Convention on the Rights of the Child. Available at http://www.ohchr.org/en/professionalinterest/pages/crc.aspx (retrieved 12 March 2015).
67. Unicef (n.d.). Fact sheet: A summary of the rights under the Convention on the Rights of the Child. Available at http://www.unicef.org/crc/files/Rights_overview.pdf (retrieved 12 March 2015).
68. Wikipedia (n.d.). Convention on the Rights of the Child. Available at http://www.en.wikipedia.org/wiki/Convention_on_the_Rights_of_the_Child (retrieved 31 March 2015).
69. Department of Health (2012). National Framework to Improve Mental Health and Wellbeing. Available at https://www.gov.uk/government/publications/national-framework-to-improve-mental-health-and-wellbeing (retrieved 1 April 2015).
70. Department of Health (2004). National Service Framework: Children, young people and maternity services. Available at https://www.gov.uk/government/publications/national-service-framework-children-young-people-and-maternity-services (retrieved 1 April 2015).
71. Newnes, C. (2005). Constructing the service user. *Clinical Psychology, 50,* 16–19.
72. Kramer, T. L., Phillips, S. D., Hargis, M. B., Miller, T. L., Burns, B. J. & Robbins, J. M. (2004). Disagreement between parent and adolescent reports of functional impairment. *Journal of Child Psychology and Psychiatry and Allied Disciplines, 45,* 248–259.

73. Russell, P., Hey, C. & Linnell, R. (2012). A qualitative exploration of Child Clinical Psychologists' understanding of user involvement. *Clinical Child Psychology and Psychiatry, 17,* 246–265.
74. Valios, N. (2002). Children in charge. *Community Care,* 28 February 2002, pp. 32–33.
75. Browne, B. W. (2005). Imagine Chicago: Cultivating hope and imagination. In C. Newnes & N. Radcliffe (Eds) *Making and Breaking Children's Lives* (pp. 151–167). Ross-on-Wye: PCCS Books. See: www.imaginechicago.org
76. Baritz, L. (1960). *The Servants of Power: A history of the use of social science in American industry.* Middletown, CT: Wesleyan University Press.
77. See Newnes, Chapter 13, this volume.
78. Hanson, H. (1996). 'Mill girls' and 'mine boys': The cultural meanings of migrant labour. *Social History, 21* (2) 160–179.
79. Newnes, C. (2015). *Inscription, Diagnosis and Deception in the Mental Health Industry: How Psy governs us all.* Basingstoke: Palgrave Macmillan.
80. Scott, R. & Meehan, G. (1972). Think about the children [Song recorded by Richie Havens]. On *The Great Blind Degree.* New York: Stormy Forest Records (1972).

Chapter 2
Constructing innocence and risk as a rationale for intervention

Melissa Burkett

Sexualisation has come to be recognised as a significant social problem in the Anglophone West, with an abundance of academic, non-academic and news media publications in the last decade detailing the potential psychological, emotional, physical, sexual and developmental risks and harms facing children – and in particular girls – as a result of their (premature and improper) exposure to an increasingly sexualised consumer and popular culture. Perceived to be innocent victims of the hyper-sexualised modern world, protection of the at-risk, vulnerable (girl) child is deemed paramount. Of course, such discourses of childhood protection and innocence are nothing new: there is a veritable history of panics and crises associated with the plight of childhood innocence – and of *female* innocence and moral purity more specifically. However, the problems and symptoms of modern society are perceived to be far worse in this 'age of anxiety'[1] in which children and young people occupy a particularly sacred and important place, and are positioned as being considerably at risk of an array of potential threats and harms to their wellbeing. This chapter highlights how the risks and harms perceived to be facing the young and innocent in the modern world (as a result of sexualisation) reflect, and rely heavily on, historical, ideological and adult social constructions of childhood, innocence, risk, vulnerability and moral purity. It is through the constant deployment and reiteration of these social constructs and the long-held ideological assumptions associated with them that a sexualisation crisis has appeared in recent times and has fast gained traction and widespread support for its eradication, primarily through calls for the urgent protection of, and intervention into, the lives of the young in order to (ironically) fix and prevent their premature and improper sexualisation.

Constructing the sexualisation crisis and the 'at risk' (girl) child

I will first outline how sexualisation has emerged as a contemporary social problem of epidemic proportions in the Anglophone West, discussing how various discourses – academic and otherwise – have combined to construct the prematurely and improperly sexualised (girl) child in dire need of protection and intervention. The term 'sexualisation' in its current form appears to stem from concerns regarding child sexual abuse in the United States in the 1970s, with UK scholar Robbie Duschinsky noting its shift from 'a specialised clinical term', in which it was used 'to refer to a liminal zone between sexual abuse and normal family life', into a term used to denote the mal-socialisation of a child or young person, becoming an important and pervasive social problem in the early 1980s.[2] From there, the term has been employed in a proliferation of discourses to refer to a process in which children and young people experience maladaptive and psychopathological outcomes as a result of prematurely internalising and embodying a notably 'adult' sexuality before they are believed to be developmentally ready.

Critical child sexuality and sexualisation scholars Gail Hawkes and Danielle Egan differentiate between conceptualisations of 'proper' and 'improper' sexualisation that are utilised in sexualisation discourses, whereby the former constitutes a key component of 'the discourse of development, a staged acquisition of approved knowledge from external (adult) sources'.[3] The latter form of sexualisation, by contrast, is *improper* because, as Hawkes and Egan note, it 'derives from unsanctioned sources, or, worse, from within the imagination or experience of the young'.[4] Thus, as a result of their developmental inadequacies, children can fall victim to improper and premature sexualisation via an internalisation of a notably 'adult' world around them. What eventuates as a result of a child's improper and premature sexualisation is an all-encompassing transformation of a state of (perceived) childhood innocence and moral purity into a remarkably fixed new identity that is deemed damaged and pathological, and which generates ongoing, long-term negative effects over the course of the child or young person's life.

Concerns about the state of modern childhood, which contributed significantly to sexualisation being granted the status of a significant social problem in the Anglophone West, stem from the backlash against child beauty pageants and the marketing of cosmetics for girls in the United States in the 1980s, both of which generated concerns regarding the destruction of childhood innocence – of a perceived normal and natural childhood – through the imposition of notably adult appearance and behaviours.[5] From there texts emerged on the problem of sexualisation, employing a 'moral reading of childhood' and deploying 'expert' commentary from those working in the disciplines of child development, education and psychology.[6] The start of a new century saw the proliferation of sexualisation as a key issue in media and public discourse, and girls – rather than patriarchy, capitalism and consumer culture – became the unit or object of analysis and key focal point in, at times, highly disparaging comments that typically focused on a girl's appearance or behaviour that was deemed distasteful, amoral and crossing the boundaries of what is perceived to be appropriate for a (respectable girl) child and for an adult.[7]

In the US, the *Report of the APA Task Force on the Sexualization of Girls* was released by the American Psychological Association (APA) in 2007 and fast gained doctrinal status as it appeared in an array of news media publications and public and academic debates, further prompting an array of academic and non-academic work, governmental inquiries and reports, and calls for the prevention of, and intervention into, the lives of children and young people.[8] Stakeholders from a range of different areas (e.g. public health, education, developmental psychology, parenting groups) have consequently engaged in the development of various programmes, measures and policy mandates to combat the pervasive and widespread effects of the problem of sexualisation. As risk theorist Deborah Lupton has noted, these 'expert knowledges … embedded within organisational contexts and often mediated through the mass media, are central to the construction and publicising of risk'.[9]

According to the oft-cited APA report, exposure to age-inappropriate media and cultural artefacts has the effect of impairing the 'mental functions and cognitive processes necessary' for normative development.[10] The report presented what was believed to be extensive evidence of the negative effects of sexualisation on girls, including low self-esteem, anxiety and depression, body image and eating disorders, cognitive and emotional deficiencies, gender and sexual developmental abnormalities, the increased risk of sexualised violence, and poor educational and academic achievement.[11] Evidence presented in the report, however, has been criticised for being considerably biased (towards negative effects), for drawing unsubstantiated conclusions (in particular through its reliance on findings collected from studies exploring other phenomena such as 'self-objectification'), and for citing almost all of its evidence from past studies involving young *adult* women attending colleges in the US.[12]

Despite its limitations and dubious omissions, however, the thesis put forth in the APA report has since taken on 'truth' status with a particular taken-for-granted 'reality' of sexualisation and the 'at-risk' girl being constructed. Following the report, psychologists and other 'experts' on sexualisation have continued to argue the apparent links between sexualisation and an array of negative physical and mental health outcomes, despite there being little to no actual research that has found any direct links. Research designed to *directly* measure and document sexualisation is also gaining traction in the psychological sciences. In some research particular measures have been devised and employed to study the impact of sexualisation on individual minds and bodies, including 'internalised sexualisation',[13] the 'Sexualising Behaviours Scale' (designed to examine the extent to which females engage in 'self-sexualising behaviour'[14]), and the 'Enjoyment of Sexualisation Scale'.[15]

As Foucault has surmised, expert knowledges are crucial to governmentality and the construction of subjectivity: they construct particular norms – through the process of normalisation – through which the individual is to be governed.[16] The psychological sciences and the research conducted within this field are pivotal to the construction and imposition of particular disciplinary techniques or technologies designed to measure, observe and intervene, and for the construction of specific advice and guidelines by which individuals are to be judged, compared and managed.[17] Through these processes, 'risk is problematised, rendered calculable and governable'[18] and particular individuals 'are identified as at risk or high risk, requiring particular forms of knowledges and interventions … which are configured using the data derived from surveillance technologies and managed by a diverse range of agencies and from a range of sites'.[19]

The politics of policy and intervention

British and Australian discourses on sexualisation have followed a similar trajectory to those in the US, though they emerged later. Jenkins and Chritcher have noted how 'domestic constituencies' are generally necessary for discourses regarding social problems to be transplanted from one location to another.[20,21] Thus, as Duschinsky further elaborates, 'a shared mobilisation of discourses on sexualisation' occurs when there are 'equivalent socio-structural issues in both settings'.[22] This is the case in the US, Britain and Australia, all of which are facing challenging social and economic times, and have, over the period of the last two decades in particular, experienced an increasingly conservative influence in the social and political spheres. Such socio-structural and cultural similarities have provided the impetus for sexualisation discourses to become naturalised and for the problem to have developed into a crisis of epidemic proportions.

In this context of social, economic and political instability and anxiety:

> incidents gain momentum, turning into dramatic public debates at salient political points in time and when cherished values are seen to be threatened by a group of identifiable people, or the 'evil Other', who need to be stopped. The process causes communal anxiety.[23]

Utilising Foucault's conceptualisation of technologies of power, Robinson argues that 'these discourses are mobilised by right-wing politicians and moral entrepreneurs to instigate a moral panic at critical points in time, in order to reassert conservative values within a heteronormative social order'.[24]

In the context of the sexualisation crisis, British Conservative Party leader David Cameron promised that, if elected, he would make certain that 'our children get a childhood' and that he would 'free' children of 'creepy' and 'inappropriate sexualisation'[25,26] which was robbing them of their childhood, arguing that 'it's about remembering the simple pleasures of our own childhood – and making sure our children can enjoy them too'.[27] Indeed, as critical sexuality scholars Jackson and Scott have noted, 'fears for children tend to be expressed through the idiom of children robbed of their childhood'.[28] Through the deployment of notions of childhood innocence and moral purity during a time of social and economic crisis, Cameron successfully mobilised sexualisation and authoritarian discourses to justify a conservative political, economic and moral campaign that would help to '[Put] Britain Back on Her Feet'.[29] Cameron effectively invoked the neoliberal tenets of (gendered) responsibility (i.e. 'by getting Britain "back on *her* feet", free of "*her*" debt and of "*her*" sexual/moral dissolution'), so integral to sexualisation discourses, to justify the scaling back of the welfare state. The sexualisation crisis, in effect, 'was headlined as the centre of the Coalition government policy on families and children'.[30]

Prior to Cameron's run for office, public and media discourse in the UK had been establishing a legacy of panic about the 'tarnished ideal of childhood'[31] and the raising of a 'generation of damaged girls'[32] in a modern, commercial world. The *Good Childhood Inquiry*[33] set forth the argument that advances in technology had resulted in a toxic state of childhood, with catastrophic effects on a child's social, cognitive and emotional development. Former Prime Minister Gordon Brown and his Labour government commissioned the Byron Review – *Safer Children in a Digital World*[34] – in 2007, which was followed by a more critical and independent assessment of *The Impact of the Commercial World on Children's Wellbeing* published in 2009.[35] Upon his election, Cameron and his Coalition government commissioned the Chief Executive of the Mothers' Union in Britain, Reg Bailey, to conduct a new review of the sexualisation of children, resulting in the highly criticised *Bailey Review of the Commercialisation and Sexualisation of Childhood* (also known as the *Letting Children Be Children* report) released in 2011.[36] This came less than a year after the release of UK 'celebrity psychologist' Linda Papadopoulos' Home Office report, the *Sexualisation of Young People Review*,[37] commissioned by the former Labour government (and which was also subjected to intense criticism for its flawed representations of the sexualisation crisis and its allegedly extensive 'evidence' of the harms facing children – and in particular girls).

Despite these flawed reports, and the even more flawed public and media commentary on sexualisation that accompanied them, conservative measures designed to restrict the rights of the child in the name of protection prevailed. For example, parallelling the spread of conservative abstinence education policy in the US during the Bush era, the UK context also witnessed increased calls for, and political intervention into, compulsory sex education policy – with renewed calls for a focus on abstinence.[38] The *Bailey Review* also recommended strict regulations to further preserve childhood innocence through the censorship and restriction of certain forms of media and advertising deemed too 'sexualised' and 'adult' for children.[39]

Coinciding with the regulations suggested in the *Bailey Review* was the *Let Girls Be Girls* campaign instigated by influential UK parenting website Mumsnet which, through its powerful lobbying and online activism, called for the strict censorship and regulation of the marketing of products deemed to instigate premature and improper sexualisation in girls. (This campaign was also publicly supported by former Prime Minister Gordon Brown at the time.[40])

In a similar vein to the UK sociopolitical context, Australian Prime Minister Kevin Rudd in 2008 also publicly expressed his concerns regarding childhood sexualisation and the need to protect childhood innocence during the heated public debates regarding an art exhibition featuring a photograph of a nude prepubescent girl.[41] The public protests against artist Bill Henson's exhibit and its improper sexualisation of an innocent (girl) child led to it being raided and closed by police. This incident and the concomitant responses to it can be situated in the context of growing unease, anxiety and concern in the Australian context regarding the sexualisation of children, in particular following the publication in 2006 of two damning – but subsequently highly criticised – reports by independent public policy think tank the Australia Institute, entitled *Corporate Paedophilia* and *Letting Children Be Children: Stopping the Sexualisation of Children in Australia*,[42,43] both of which facilitated intense public, media and academic debate about the status of modern childhood in an increasingly risky and harmful commercialised and sexualised culture. These reports further prompted a Senate inquiry into the 'sexualisation of children in the contemporary media environment'.[44] Further, similar to the UK context, in Australia online activism against sexualisation has also gained traction since 2007 (around the time of the release of the APA report) with mother-of-two Julie Gale founding the no-longer-active website Kids Free 2B Kids, and Melinda Tankard Reist founding Collective Shout (www.collectiveshout.org), both of which sought to challenge the commercialisation and sexualisation of children (the latter focusing more so on girls) through their online petitions and calls for censorship, protection and intervention in the name of preserving childhood – but predominantly young female – innocence.

In these sexualisation debates in the political and media fields, discourses of parental rights, children's rights and childhood innocence have been strategically mobilised in an effort to reinstate conservative values, and to call for and justify intrusive interventions into the lives of young people, and the censorship and eradication of external influences deemed harmful to their normative development. With regard to the Henson exhibit more specifically, and situating it more broadly in the context of the sexualisation crisis, it is the child's *susceptibility* to external danger and corruption – the *potential* for their innocence and purity to be compromised – and for their dormant sexuality to consequently become prematurely and improperly awakened, that drive concerns and calls for protection and intervention.

Following highly publicised incidents such as these, pressure groups and 'experts' hold great sway in pushing for urgent reform and intervention – legal, political, educational and so on – as seen with the highly successful Mumsnet petitions in the UK context, and the strong influence of Australian online activist communities like Collective

Shout and Kids Free 2B Kids. The panic expressed by these stakeholders in the protection of childhood innocence is, however, not about the sexualisation of girls *per se*; rather it is facilitated by a yearning for a return to a state of perceived innocence for *certain* children and females – notably those of the middle class.[45] This is made abundantly clear in Garbarino's highly influential text *Raising Children in a Socially Toxic Environment*, which played a significant role in spurring heated discussion about the moral corruption of childhood in the US as a result of a 'toxic' social and cultural environment. In it, he argued:

> An environment is becoming increasingly socially toxic when we observe an erosion of *middle-class* childhood. Childhood is the measuring stick for assessing social change [italics mine].[46]

Thus, when the norms of middle-class childhood – and more specifically middle-class girlhood – appear to be undergoing a process of contamination via sexualised culture we can be certain that we have a significant problem on our hands, and that the best efforts of policy makers, politicians, the 'Psy' industry and other normalising and moralising disciplines will be put forth to try to investigate, prevent and intervene.

Constructing normative childhood innocence

As mentioned, in contemporary sexualisation narratives, the natural developmental process as posited in traditional psychological theories can be threatened and corrupted by external forces, whether that is by an adult, the media or another aspect of culture; that is, sexualised objects that are already imbued with *adult* meaning work through a process of osmosis when they encounter children.[47] Subsequently, as Egan and Hawkes posited, 'corrupt causes are said to incite a form of sexuality that, under "normal" circumstances, would have been either dormant or absent altogether'.[48] For anti-sexualisation advocates, 'sexuality should be an "independent island nation" untainted by the avarice of corporations and free of cultural influence'.[49] Thus, 'the implicit assumption is that sexual innocence and, by implication, childhood is a state of *nature* which stands *outside* of culture and capitalism' (my italics).[50] It is this interference of *nature*, and premature awakening of 'dormant or absent' sexuality – a 'robbing of childhood', through the contamination of the child's mind and body by 'exposure' to external 'adult' forces – that is of great concern in sexualisation narratives. This can be seen most clearly in ongoing debates regarding the timing and content of sex education in the UK, US and Australian contexts, which have intensified in light of the sexualisation panic.

In sexualisation narratives, including those deployed in formal reports, the child and childhood are often left undefined, relying instead on the audience's commonsense knowledge and understanding regarding what a 'child' and 'childhood' are. The assumptions, claims and key arguments integral to sexualisation narratives rest on the ideal of the innocent child, which has strong historical roots in the Anglophone West. Indeed, childhood innocence as a natural state has been key to a veritable legacy of sexual and moral panics regarding the potential sexual and moral corruption of youth, including the 'purity' and 'sexual hygiene' movements of the nineteenth century, and more recent panics over the potential risks and dangers of novels, comic books, television and of course most recently the internet.[51] These panics have provided the impetus for intensive surveillance and regulation of childhood and youth sexuality to this day. Thus, contemporary fears regarding the potential corruption of children and young people are steeped in history in the Anglophone West, and we tend to draw on these historical legacies and the emotions (e.g. fear, anxiety, disgust) they invoke when we are faced with new and emerging social and moral problems, such as that of sexualisation.[52]

As historians and sociologists have argued alongside extensive evidence, however, the ideal of the innocent child in need of protection is a relatively recent social and cultural construct, with specific ties to Judeo-Christian and bourgeois Victorian culture.[53] Literary critic James Kincaid has also identified links between our modern obsession with childhood innocence and Romantic and post-Romantic period philosophy in which the child is 'free of adult corruptions'.[54] The contemporary institutional surveillance and protection of children has also been a key part of capitalist culture, with 'family and educational institutions' in the mid-nineteenth century called upon 'to preserve [childhood] innocence and purity en route to adulthood'.[55] The deployment of developmental psychological discourses and discourses of child protection concomitantly resulted in greater 'expert' surveillance and intervention of migrant and working-class children and families who were deemed to be more at risk.[56] Deviation from the strictly defined and culturally (note: white, middle-class) constructed parameters of normative childhood development and innocence therefore resulted in the pathologisation of lower, working-class children and intensive intervention at the state level.[57] As Nikolas

Rose notes, this was all done to 'safeguard' the child 'from physical, sexual and moral danger, to ensure its "normal" development'.[58]

The work of Sigmund Freud disrupted long-held Victorian assumptions and ideals about the asexual and innocent child, and other developments of ideas in the areas of sexology and psychology in the twentieth century saw some further recognition of the sexuality of children.[59] However, this served to increase regulation in order to ensure the curtailment of 'abnormal' or 'deviant' sexual behaviours.[60] In the late twentieth and early twenty-first centuries we witnessed the rise of 'risk anxiety' in the Anglophone West, with children typically at the centre of panics.[61] Ironically, contemporary risk discourses invoke a 'nostalgia for an imagined past in which children played safely throughout a carefree childhood', the reality of which is quite different, as for some time now children have been the subject of moral panics resulting in increased surveillance.[62] However, whereas in the past children were governed by protective discourses, these discourses have today been fused together with risk anxiety, fostering an increasing preoccupation with preventative measures and 'a need for constant vigilance in order to anticipate and guard against potential threats to children's well-being'.[63]

The 'Ophelia industry' and the contaminated Other

Sexualisation narratives go deeper than simply reproducing traditional ideologies regarding childhood innocence. In positioning the sexualised girl as deviant, sexualisation narratives draw on historical and long-standing ideologies of race, class, age and gender in which the reputation and respectability of white, middle-class girls serve as regulatory or disciplinary technologies.[64] The contemporary problem of sexualisation can therefore be historically situated in the context of other modern, Western crises of childhood, and in particular girlhood, in which notions of health and normality have been constructed and mobilised as part of an increasing surveillance and regulation of the (girl) child.

Towards the end of the nineteenth century, as a result of the increased participation of young females in the modern and public spheres of work, education, sport and leisure, the concept of girlhood evolved, with specific physical and mental health issues facing the girl population deemed important for observation and intervention.[65] In dominant medical discourses at the time denoting the risks associated with adolescence, and more specifically puberty, girls were deemed 'victims' of a certain 'biological vulnerability' which coincided with an array of 'symptoms' needing intervention in order for the girl to achieve good health.[66] These 'new models of healthy girlhood', which were established in the late Victorian era, were not straightforwardly imposed by external influences but, rather, accorded responsibility to the girl herself, who was required to ensure that she properly ascribed to the 'rules of health'.[67] These rules were increasingly outlined and disseminated in advice literature prepared by a burgeoning group of 'experts' including medical professionals, teachers, journalists and writers, and so on. These disciplinary techniques designed to control and regulate the body are commonly concealed in discourses of risk and protection in which individuals are provided with advice and instruction on how they should best conduct their lives.[68]

This 'preoccupation with prevention' and intervention into the lives of girls more specifically is concomitantly linked with the continued expansion and power of the 'Ophelia industry', which contributes to the 'psychological knowledge constituting girlhood … assist[ing] in the production of the new self-inventing, neoliberal girl subject'.[69] This industry and its knowledges underpin and facilitate neoliberal and conservative social, moral, economic and political agendas, like some of those discussed earlier in this chapter. Discourses of risk and protection essentially serve 'as no more than the conservation of a pre-existing purity, [and] as the cover for a covert training and normalisation through the control over the environment and choices of minors'.[70]

In her critical text on girlhood in the modern world, Gonick reflected on how the Shakespearean character of Ophelia has been utilised in past and present crises about girlhood to represent social and moral concern for the girl deemed to be at-risk and vulnerable.[71] She notes how in the nineteenth century Ophelia was mobilised during the hysteria crisis and also appeared to symbolise Hall's conceptualisation of the adolescent girl in his work on normative forms of girlhood, in which he drew attention to the gendered, chaotic state of adolescence during which time it is girls who are perceived to suffer the most and who are consequently in dire need of psychological and medical intervention. This 'biological vulnerability' of the girl has continued into more modern-day crises of girlhood which have spawned the self-help and parenting advice market with, for example, Mary Pipher's 1994 text *Reviving Ophelia: Saving the selves of adolescent girls*, in which she argues that girls encounter a 'crisis of self-esteem' in adolescence – similar to Hall's arguments – that has dire pathological outcomes on their normative development into 'healthy' adulthood.[72] Discourses of girls' vulnerability have therefore flourished as part of an agenda to 'fix' the at-risk, vulnerable girl and, as Gonick further noted, this has facilitated the commercialisation of the Ophelia crisis, spearheading the careers of predominantly *adult* women who have entered the market as 'experts' on the plight of girls, often reminiscing about their own (apparently) innocent and morally pure childhood and adolescence. In the current context of the sexualisation crisis, these 'experts' have contributed to a burgeoning pseudo-psychological literature on the sexualised, at-risk and vulnerable girl, with highly popular (and fear- and anxiety-provoking) titles including: *The Lolita Effect*; *What's Happening to Our Girls? Too Much, Too Soon: How our kids are over-stimulated, over-sold and over-sexed*; *Where Has My Little Girl Gone?*; *Girls Gone Skank: The sexualisation of girls in American culture*; and *So Sexy So Soon: The new sexualised childhood and what parents can do to protect their kids*.

As mentioned, often harsh and emotion-driven classist language is employed in these texts in descriptions about sexualised girls who are perceived to have transgressed moral and class boundaries; such language invokes bourgeois stereotypes of the working-class prostitute, for example.[73,74] Through invoking strong affective responses to potential threats to the moral purity and innocence of middle-class girls as a result of perceived class contagion, sexualisation narratives generate widespread fear, concern and even panic at the changing social and moral world. Indeed, social class 'plays a central role in the regulation of femininity and the production of Otherness'.[75] Thus, it is the figure of the *white, middle-class girl child* and the potential for her innocence to be contaminated by the amoral working-class Other – who is associated with 'overly sexual displays of low culture' – that prompts the strongest emotional responses in the Anglophone West.[76] In this sense, as Egan and Hawkes have argued, classed boundaries are being redrawn and policed between low- and high-status culture, with substantive discursive and practical efforts being deployed to prevent the 'infiltration of working class feminine sexuality' into what is perceived to be the 'uncontaminated domain' of middle-class femininity.[77]

As Fischer has argued, 'there is no universal agreement as to what constitutes sexually immoral behaviour', and 'what gets defined as moral and immoral is arbitrary in a historical sense'.[78] In modern society it is not so much the *acts* that are engaged in that are considered immoral or morally corrupt but rather the *identity* of those who engage in the behaviour; deviance is typically conceptualised in terms of *identities* rather than *acts*.[79] Thus, it is not the sexualised behaviours *per se* that are deemed deviant in sexualisation narratives, but rather it is the *child* – the young *middle-class girl* – engaging in such behaviour or displaying such an appearance, considered to be unfeminine, lower class or too adult, who is considered deviant and amoral.[80,81,82,83] In this sense, terms like 'slut' and 'skank', commonly used in sexualisation narratives, refer more to the identity of the individual rather than the behaviour or act being performed or engaged in. Here, the 'slut', as a 'mythic figure' and folk devil, 'marks the boundary of gendered and sexual acceptability'[84] and serves as a cautionary tale for respectable middle-class girls. Through invoking a folk devil – the morally contaminated and polluted Other – the innocent and morally pure girl is once again constructed as in need of protection and intervention so as to ensure she does not follow the same route should she be prematurely and improperly sexualised. Thus, the girl 'is positioned as a risk assemblage in a web of surveillance, monitoring, measurement and expert advice that requires constant work on her part'.[85]

Concluding comments

In contemporary sexualisation discourses, it is the risks posed to normative sexual and moral development that form the foundations of calls for the imposition of protection and intervention into the lives of the (girl) child so as to ensure the 'present and future reproductive, social, and economic life of the nation'.[86] Through the invocation of themes of purity, innocence, risk and vulnerability, sexualisation discourses construct sexuality and sexual knowledge as forms of 'cultural contagion, coming from outside the (middle-class) home, from which girls need protection by parents and other social authorities'.[87] Consequently, 'the result is a justification for the social and self-regulation of *young female subjects* as inadequate economic, social, and (hetero) sexual choice-making agents' (my italics).[88]

As Duschinsky further notes, there are three areas of neoliberal decision-making subjectivity: political consent, sexual consent, and consumption and entrepreneurship.[89] Children (and girls more specifically) function *outside* of this subjectivity and therefore must be carefully moulded and 'nourished by the correct processes of training'[90] and education – through sex (or indeed abstinence) education and other policies and interventions – so as to ensure they become responsible, neoliberal subjects in the future and do not place a strain on state resources. Indeed, in modern times 'in which responsible subjectivity has become a key target of neoliberal biopolitical discourses':

> Proper childhood is also a covert training ground in *proper* choice-making, so as to stabilise the tension between the *natural* and *desirable* state of neo-liberal subjects [italics mine].[91]

This is particularly the case in sexualisation discourses as outlined in this chapter, which, through their mobilisation during times of social, economic and political anxiety and upheaval in Western Anglophone countries (as mentioned earlier), have served to justify the increased imposition of measures designed to intervene in the lives of children – and girls more specifically as they are positioned as the future of modern society – under the guise of protecting a naturalised, socially constructed and pre-existing state of innocence and moral purity.

This chapter provides a brief outline of how sexualisation has come to be regarded as a significant social problem in the Anglophone West, and how sexualisation narratives have deployed long-held historical ideologies of race, class, age and gender in an attempt to evoke strong affective responses to the potential threat sexualisation poses to childhood innocence, the moral purity of middle-class girlhood, and to the moral and social fabric of society more broadly. Through highlighting the limitations and omissions of psychological and other 'expert' discourses on sexualisation, and their reliance on unsubstantiated facts and assumptions about normative development and middle-class girls' sexuality, I hope that this chapter, along with an emerging body of literature adopting a more critical approach to sexualisation narratives, sheds further light on the underlying problems of these narratives and how their 'truth' claims can cause unintended harm by categorising children – predominantly girls – into rigid and stereotyped 'normal'/'innocent'/'moral' and 'deviant'/'contaminated'/'amoral' categories, prompting often unnecessary paternalistic surveillance and intervention into their lives.

Endnotes

1. Hollway, W. & Jefferson, T. (1997). The risk society in an age of anxiety. *British Journal of Sociology, 48*, 255–266.
2. Duschinsky, R. (2013a). The emergence of sexualization as a social problem: 1981–2010. *Social Politics, 20* (1) 137–156, pp. 139–140.
3. Hawkes, G. L. & Egan, R. D. (2008). Landscapes of erotophobia: The sexual(ized) child in the postmodern anglophone west. *Sexuality & Culture, 12*, 193–203, p. 199.
4. Ibid.

5. Duschinsky, 2013a. See note 2.
6. Ibid.
7. Duschinsky, R. (2013b). Sexualisation: A state of injury. *Theory & Psychology, 23* (3) 351–370.
8. American Psychological Association (2007). *Report of the APA Task Force on the Sexualization of Girls*. Washington, DC: American Psychological Association.
9. Lupton, D. (1999). *Risk: Key ideas*. London: Routledge.
10. APA, 2007, p. 19. See note 8.
11. Ibid.
12. Lerum, K. & Dworkin, S. L. (2009). 'Bad girls rule': An interdisciplinary feminist commentary on the report of the APA Task Force on the Sexualization of Girls. *Journal of Sex Research, 46* (4) 250–263.
13. McKenney, S. J. & Bigler, R. S. (2014). Internalized sexualization and its relation to sexualized appearance, body surveillance, and body shame among early adolescent girls. *The Journal of Early Adolescence* [online first]. Available at http://jea.sagepub.com/content/early/2014/10/31/0272431614556889.abstract (retrieved 8 April 2015).
14. Nowatzki, J. & Morry, M. M. (2009). Women's intentions regarding, and acceptance of, self-sexualizing behaviour. *Psychology of Women Quarterly*, 33 (1) 95–107.
15. Liss, M., Erchull, M. J. & Ramsey, L. R. (2011). Empowering or oppressing? Development and exploration of the Enjoyment of Sexualisation Scale. *Personality and Social Psychology Bulletin*, 37 (1), 55–68.
16. Foucault, M. (1991). Governmentality. In G. Burchell, C. Gordon & P. Miller (Eds) *The Foucault Effect: Studies in governmentality* (pp. 87–104). Hemel Hempstead: Harvester Wheatsheaf.
17. Rose, N. (1998). *Inventing Our Selves: Psychology, power, and personhood*. Cambridge, UK: Cambridge University Press.
18. Lupton, 1999, p. 117. See note 9.
19. Ibid.
20. Jenkins, P. (1998). *Moral Panic: Changing concepts of the child molester in modern America*. New Haven, CT: Yale University Press.
21. Critcher, C. (2003). *Moral Panics and the Media*. Buckingham: Open University Press.
22. Duschinsky, 2013a, p. 145. See note 2.
23. Robinson, K. H. (2008). In the name of 'childhood innocence': A discursive exploration of the moral panic associated with childhood and sexuality. *Cultural Studies Review, 14* (2) 113–129.
24. Ibid.
25. *Daily Mail* (2010a). Cameron attacks 'creepy sexualisation' of children. Available at http://www.dailymail.co.uk/news/article-385711/Cameron-attacks-creepy-sexualisation-children.html (retrieved 8 April 2015).
26. *Daily Mail* (2010b). Tories will clamp down on 'sexualisation' of children, vows David. Available at http://www.dailymail.co.uk/news/article-1251908/David-Cameron-Tories-clamp-sexualisation-children.html (retrieved 8 April 2015).
27. BBC (2010). Stop sexualising children, says David Cameron. BBC News, February 18 2010. Available at http://news.bbc.co.uk/2/hi/8521403.stm (retrieved 8 April 2015).
28. Jackson, S. & Scott, S. (2010). *Theorizing Sexuality*. Maidenhead: Open University Press.
29. Cameron, D. (2009). Putting Britain back on her feet: Address to the Conservative Party Conference. Available at http://www.conservatives.com/News/Speeches/2009/10/

David_Cameron_Putting_Britain_back_on_her_feet.aspx (retrieved 8 April 2015).
30. Duschinsky, 2013b. See note 7.
31. Kehily, M. J. (2012). Contextualising the sexualisation of girls debate: Innocence, experience and young female sexuality. *Gender and Education, 24* (3) 255–268.
32. Womack, S. (2007). The generation of 'damaged' girls. *Telegraph*, 2 February 2007. Available at http://www.telegraph.co.uk/news/health/1543203/The-generation-of-damaged-girls.html (retrieved 8 April 2015).
33. Children's Society (2007). *Good Childhood Inquiry: Reflections on childhood-lifestyle*. London: GfK Social Research.
34. Byron, T. (2008). *Safer Children in a Digital World: The report of the Byron Review 2008*. London: DCSF.
35. Department for Children, Schools and Families (2009). *The Impact of the Commercial World on Children's Wellbeing*. London: DCSF.
36. Bailey, R. (2011). *Letting Children Be Children: Report of an independent review of the commercialisation and sexualisation of childhood*. London: Department for Education.
37. Papadopoulos, L. (2010). *Sexualisation of Young People Review*. London: Home Office.
38. Duschinsky, 2013a. See note 2.
39. Bailey, 2011. See note 36.
40. Bragg, S., Buckingham, D., Russell, R. & Willett, R. (2011). Too much, too soon? Children, 'sexualisation' and consumer culture. *Sex Education, 11* (3) 279–292.
41. Hawkes & Egan, 2008. See note 3.
42. Rush, E. & La Nauze, A. (2006a). *Corporate Paedophilia: Sexualisation of children in Australia*. Canberra: The Australia Institute.
43. Rush, E. & La Nauze, A. (2006b). *Letting Children be Children: Stopping the Sexualisation of Children in Australia*. Canberra: The Australia Institute.
44. Senate Standing Committee on Environment, Communications and the Arts (2008). *Sexualisation of Children in the Contemporary Media*. Canberra: Senate Printing Unit, Parliament House.
45. Egan, R. D. (2013). *Becoming Sexual: A critical appraisal of the sexualization of girls*. Malden, MA: Polity.
46. Garbarino, J. (1995). *Raising Children in a Socially Toxic Environment*. San Francisco: Jossey-Bass.
47. Egan, R. D. & Hawkes, G. L. (2008a). Endangered girls and incendiary objects: Unpacking the discourse on sexualisation. *Sexuality & Culture, 12*, 291–311.
48. Ibid.
49. Egan, 2013. See note 45.
50. Ibid.
51. Egan & Hawkes, 2008a. See note 47.
52. Egan, 2013. See note 45.
53. Jackson, S. & Scott, S. (2010). *Theorizing Sexuality*. Maidenhead: Open University Press.
54. Kincaid, J. (1998). *Erotic Innocence: The culture of child molesting*. Durham, NC: Duke University Press, pp. 14–15.
55. Evans, D. T. (1993). *Sexual Citizenship: The material construction of sexualities*. London: Routledge, p. 211.
56. Egan & Hawkes, 2008a. See note 47.
57. Rose, N. (1989). *Governing the Soul: The shaping of the private self*. London: Free Association Books.
58. Ibid. p. 123.

59. Egan, R. D. & Hawkes, G. L. (2010). Childhood sexuality, normalization and the social hygiene movement in the Anglophone West, 1900-1935. *Social History of Medicine, 23* (1) 56-78.
60. Jackson, S. & Scott, S. (2010). *Theorizing Sexuality*. Maidenhead: Open University Press.
61. Ibid.
62. Ibid. p. 105.
63. Ibid. p. 106.
64. Egan, 2013. See note 45.
65. Marland, H. (2013). *Health and Girlhood in Britain, 1874-1920*. London: Palgrave Macmillan.
66. Ibid.
67. Ibid.
68. Rose, 1989. See note 57.
69. Gonick, M. (2006). Between 'girl power' and 'reviving Ophelia': Constituting the neoliberal girl subject. *NWSA Journal, 18* (2) 1-23, p. 18.
70. Duschinsky, 2013b, p. 363. See note 7.
71. Gonick, 2006. See note 69.
72. Pipher, M. (1994). *Reviving Ophelia: Saving the selves of adolescent girls*. New York: Grosset/Putnam.
73. Egan, 2013. See note 45.
74. Egan & Hawkes, 2008a. See note 47.
75. Walkerdine, V. (1998). *Daddy's Girl: Young girls and popular culture*. Cambridge, MA: Harvard University Press, p. 171.
76. Egan & Hawkes (2008a), p. 306. See note 47.
77. Ibid.
78. Fischer, N. (2006). Purity and pollution: Sex as a moral discourse. In S. Seidman, N. Fischer & C. Meeks (Eds) *Handbook of the New Sexuality Studies* (pp. 56-63). New York: Routledge, p. 56.
79. Papadopoulos, L. (2010). *Sexualisation of Young People Review*. London: Home Office.
80. Duschinsky, 2013b. See note 7.
81. Egan, 2013. See note 45.
82. Egan & Hawkes, 2008a. See note 47.
83. Kehily, M. J. (2012). Contextualising the sexualisation of girls debate: Innocence, experience and young female sexuality. *Gender and Education, 24* (3) 255-268.
84. Egan, 2013, p. 31. See note 45.
85. Lupton, 1999, p. 121. See note 9.
86. Duschinsky, 2013b, p. 364. See note 7.
87. Ibid. p. 363.
88. Ibid.
89. Ibid.
90. Ibid. p. 362.
91. Ibid.

Chapter 3
The Stolen Generations: The forced removal of First Peoples children in Australia

Pat Dudgeon, Carmen Cubillo and Abigail Bray

> I was at the post office with my Mum and Auntie [and cousin]. They put us in the police ute and said they were taking us to Broome. They put the mums in there as well. But when we'd gone [about 10 miles] they stopped, and threw the mothers out of the car. We jumped on our mothers' backs, crying, trying not to be left behind. But the policemen pulled us off and threw us back in the car. They pushed the mothers away and drove off, while our mothers were chasing the car, running and crying after us. We were screaming in the back of that car. When we got to Broome they put me and my cousin in the Broome lock-up. We were only 10 years old. We were in the lock-up for two days waiting for the boat to Perth.[1]

In 2008 the governments of Australia and Canada offered separate but similar apologies to the Stolen Generations of First Peoples who had been forcible removed as children from their parents, home, communities, culture, language and land since the late eighteenth century. These government apologies secured a hegemonic belief that the removal of children, and the overt oppression of First Peoples, had ended. For example, Mills claims in *Studies in Australian Political Rhetoric*: 'All of the wrongdoing behaviours have now ceased, and the former official sanction for them has been withdrawn.'[2] However, in Australia in 2015 a Gunnedah group, Grandmothers Against Removals, are seeking to draw attention to an *increased* removal of First Peoples children from their families.[3] And in Canada in 2015 a new wave of removals termed the 'Millennium Scoop' has followed the 'Sixties Scoop', an intensive wave of removals from the 1950s to the 1990s.[4] In both white settler nations the removal of First Peoples children from their families and communities continues a practice that both nations, after pressure from extensive First Peoples lobbying, have all but admitted is an act of genocide. In both nations *unprecedented* numbers of children are now being taken. In Australia and Canada white child protection discourses continue to legitimate an escalation in the genocidal removal of First Peoples children.

This chapter considers the removal of Indigenous children as a global colonial and neocolonial tactic by exploring some of the historical similarities between the nations that have been named the United States of America, Canada and Australia. The history of the Australian Stolen Generations is then focused on, from the beginning of the abduction of children in the early 1900s up until 2015. The landmark 1997 report *Bringing Them Home: Report of the National Inquiry into the Separation of Aboriginal and Torres Strait Islander Children from their Families* is central to the emergence of national and international awareness of the systemic abuse of First Peoples human rights in Australia and the profound wounding of Stolen Generations.

Drawing attention to how the removal of First Peoples children is sanctioned by Western child-rearing discourses, the chapter explores how the pathologisation of Indigenous families by such discourses embeds racist stereotypes of neglectful Indigenous mothers, abusive Indigenous fathers and damaged Indigenous children as deviant Others. In this context, the Australian Indigenous mental health movement has emerged within a rising decolonisation movement founded on the principle of self-determination. Indigenous psychology in Australia, although a historically recent movement, has been at the forefront of decolonising the Western child development and child-rearing discourses which justified, and continue to justify, the removal of Indigenous children from their people.[5] The movement is also reviving and supporting culturally appropriate healing in order to strengthen and restore the social and emotional wellbeing of First Peoples damaged by generations of forced removals.

Overlapping circles of extended family lie at the heart of the lives of most Aboriginal Australians. Networks of family relationships determine day-to-day activities and shape the course of destinies. From an early age Aboriginal Australians learn who belongs to whom, where and whom they have come from, and how they should behave across a wide universe of kin. These are highly valued and integral components of Aboriginal cultural knowledge. Yet these same familial systems have been the site of repeated attacks by successive waves of Australian governments, tearing at the very heart of Aboriginal family life.[6] Removing children hurt everybody.

Various reports – such as the *Bringing Them Home Report* – have shown that in certain Australian regions, at different times, more than one in ten children were taken.[7] Not one Indigenous family has escaped the effects of forcible removal and most families have been affected over several generations. McGrath described policies for the removal of children as 'the ultimate racist act':

> It was a conscious decision to conduct state interference in this most fundamental human relationship between mother and child. The mother laboured to produce it, then suckled and nurtured it. Protectiveness, dependency and love for children are among the strongest human feelings, and the right to reproduce and nurture a basic human right. State intervention in the reproductive sphere grew out of a collective attempt to grab back the products of the white man's spilt seed for the white 'race'. In a paranoid reaction to Aboriginal women's power in Territory society, they were consequently to be denied their right to rear, influence and make decisions about their children and forced to suffer and sometimes be crushed by the psychological trauma of the loss. Lack of empathy for their plight reflected the power of racial stereotypes which assumed Aboriginal women had no feelings.[8]

Haebich's comprehensive analysis of the removal of Indigenous Australian children across the country describes this as an ongoing process that took place from colonisation to the present day.[9] The consequences of this process of forced removals are part of Indigenous identity.

It has only been in recent times that the practice has been officially recognised with the former Prime Minister Paul Keating's historic Redfern Park Speech in 1992, where, within a list of racial claims that Australia has perpetrated upon its Indigenous peoples, he stated, '*We took the children away from their mothers.*' The legacy of that practice remains today, in terms of a reduced life span, a suicide epidemic, a broad pattern of socioeconomic disadvantage and ill-health, malignant grief, and ongoing and culminative trauma. This was followed by Prime Minister Kevin Rudd's 2008 speech in Parliament which had bi-partisan endorsement.

Colonisation

Indigenous peoples are in the process of decolonisation. For many Indigenous societies, particularly in settler countries where the experience of the effects of colonisation has continued, 'reclaiming a collective identity and shared culture is critical for forging a regenerated, resistant cultural identity to challenge colonial representations that ... have justified oppressive practices that have had devastating effects on Indigenous social and emotional wellbeing'.[10] Following Smith, the term 'postcolonial' is not used here because it activates the kind of historical amnesia that lulls invader cultures into forgetting the still dynamic yet disavowed foundations of invaded nations – *complex cultural genocide*.[11] Aileen Morton-Robinson, an Indigenous Australian intellectual, has stated that the situation in Australia is very different from a postcolonial perspective, arguing that 'it is not postcolonial in the same way that India, Malaysia and Algeria can be said to be. These nations do not have a dominant white settler population. In Australia, the colonials do not go home.'[12] The term 'postcolonialism' is also inflected with a broader postmodern rejection of essentialism and, therefore, the need to reclaim a separate cultural identity. Ian Anderson, a Tasmanian Indigenous academic, critiques the theoretical condemnation of essentialism. According to Anderson, those who reject essentialism ignore the reasons why Aboriginal people use essentialism to construct identities to claim their culture back in their own ways:

> Essentialism is not an instrinsic evil. It is the product of social relations which may empower or disempower Aboriginal people. Those who wish to police Aboriginalities by disallowing essentailising identities have ignored the importance of identity as a relation of bodies, practices, past. In subverting hegemonic forms of Aboriginalism, it may be a valid strategy to re-integrate and enclose. This offers people the potential to convey of themselves as Aboriginal bodies, within an Aboriginal time and landscape.[13]

Furthermore, while for the majority of the population of Australia belonging is linked to dispossession and migration, Indigenous people have an ontological relation with the land and position all others as migrants and diasporic. Ontological belonging means that Indigenous people have a spiritual sense of belonging to land or country. Colonisation has not destroyed this relationship. Moreton-Robinson dismisses anti-essentialist concerns by proposing that such arguments are still premised on Western constructions, and are applied as universal, despite epistemological recognition of difference:

> It may be argued that to suggest an ontological relationship to describe Indigenous belonging is essentialist, or is a form of strategic essentialism because I am imputing an essence of belonging. From an Indigenous epistemology, what is essentialist is the premise upon which such criticism depends: the Western definition of the self as not unitary nor fixed. This is a form of strategic essentialism that can silence and dismiss non-Western constructions that do not define the self in the same way.[14]

This chapter, then, recognises that colonisation is continuous and practised against a people, and questions the political investment in triumphalist Enlightenment master narratives about progressive Western modernity. As Bhabha writes: 'The struggle against colonial oppression changes not only the direction of Western history, but challenges its historicist "idea" of time as a progressive, ordered whole.'[15] The term 'neocolonialism', on the other hand, captures the convergence between neoliberalism and colonialism. Neoliberalism is a hegemonic global Western ideology, which mystifies the economic and historical foundations of oppressive social relations by promoting the ideal of a heroic meritocratic individual strangely immune from the structurally entrenched inequities of late-capitalism. In the shadows of this shiny individualism are surplus populations who are being stripped of substantive rights by neoliberal austerity regimes just as they are told that poverty is an individual choice, a symptom of laziness, innate stupidity and deviance. In the depths of the shadow cast by Western individualism are the children of the First Peoples who continue to be targeted by neocolonial governments as 'at risk', not from systemic racist oppression, but from their own pathologised, criminalised and infantilised cultures, and who must, in effect, be rescued from their own people, adjusted and corrected, culturally bleached and purified, reared by the very discourses of white Western individualism that cast them as shadows. Although the discourse of neoliberal individualism is marketed as egalitarianism, it can be understood as an expansion of the politics of social Darwinism. In other words, the discourse of neoliberal egalitarian individualism masks the rise of a re-scientised racism, which diagnoses some members of the population as more or less evolved than others.[16]

Australian history can be summarised as the story of how Aboriginal peoples lost a continent and how invaders gained one. The take-over of lands included the dispossessing of the people at all levels.[17] While opponents of Aboriginal rights argue that land rights or native title will divide the nation, any study of the past reveals that from the earliest times the British set about creating boundaries and social divisions; the land and its riches were divided up in increasingly uneven portions between the newcomers and the Aboriginal people.[18] While British colonialism is the overarching background to the history of Australia, the local and individual lives of Indigenous people and how they dealt with these historical, social and political realities over the past 200 and more years has determined their identity.

According to Richard Broome, there are two preconceptions about non-Western peoples that influenced the views about Australian Aborigines held by British colonists: that of the 'savage' and that of the 'noble savage'.[19] The former was associated with Aboriginal people being perceived to be animalistic, violent, lecherous, treacherous, black, dirty and evil. The latter was a more romantic and positive view of people living as one with nature. However, overall the colonists who came to Australia held pessimistic and negative views of Aboriginal people. Regardless, the consequences of Western colonialism were disastrous for Indigenous people not only in Australia but also all over the globe.

Until recent times, Australian history has been written from a romanticised Eurocentric standpoint which minimised the violence of colonisation and celebrated the white settler as hero. If Aboriginal people were present in these histories, they were depicted as backward people who were easily pushed aside in the settlement of the country. The act of writing history has always been a political act, and past and present Australian historians have played a significant role in nation building.[20] Indigenous Australians were mostly absent from Australian histories until W.E.H. Stanner challenged this in his famous Boyer lectures in 1968, *The Great Australian Silence*.[21] Authors such as Charles Rowley, Richard Broome, Peter Biskup, Henry Reynolds and other scholars, including Aboriginal writers, started writing different and groundbreaking historical accounts that have challenged previously held historical writings on the settlement of the country. It is largely accepted nowadays that there are different perspectives of history.[22]

An acknowledgement of dominant history is warranted in this chapter, as it is only recently that the subjective and imperial roles of history as part of the colonising project have been understood and challenged. While the effects of these dominant views are still prevalent in society, the presence of previously hidden histories is now being strengthened and becoming part of the Australian national story. Considerations of how people from various oppressed cultural groups saw themselves, and the fact that they lived in a dominant racist world, have begun to enter the national narrative despite a conservative backlash. Indigenous resistances and, thereby, Indigenous views and standpoints about history have been denied, and been made absent or invisible in the discourse of Australian nationhood. Indigenous resistances have had many manifestations, and as Moreton-Robinson states:

> In our engagement with white Australian society, Indigenous people have learnt to create meaning, knowledges and living traditions under conditions not of our own choosing as strategies for our survival. Our cultural forms take account of the ambiguous existence that is the inevitable result of this engagement.[23]

Under colonialism, Indigenous peoples have struggled against a Western view of history that has excluded or distorted and denigrated them and their cultures. This is reinforced in the public institutions of life, particularly schooling and education. Indigenous scholars from other settler countries have shared this concern. Tuhiwai Smith proposed that challenging colonisers' histories is an imperative for Indigenous peoples.[24] Forcible removals of children and their subsequent effects have been a profound part of the Indigenous Australian story.[25] This chapter on the Stolen Generations of children is, therefore, part of this collective imperative to challenge colonisers' histories.

The forced removal of First Peoples children

In the nations invaded by Europe, including the countries that have been named Australia, Canada, North America, South America and India, the First Peoples children were systematically targeted by the usurping white nation, removed from their families, institutionalised, abused and exploited. In settler nations the practice of removing Indigenous children from families and communities was not only done to assimilate children but also to *disintegrate* Indigenous communities and break the relationship between Indigenous people and their environment.[26]

During the 1987 Vancouver World Conference of Indigenous Peoples' Education, similarities were discovered between the mistreatment of Coorg children in India and First Peoples children in Canada.[27] One Coorg child 'was physically tortured by his teachers for speaking Tseshaht: they pushed sewing needles through his tongue, a routine punishment for language offenders'.[28] As Haig-Brown observes, the 'elimination of language has always been a primary stage in a process of cultural genocide'.[29] *Cultural genocide begins with children.* As the Aboriginal and Torres Strait Islander Corporation of Languages submission, cited in *Bringing Them Home,* states: 'What must be remembered is that language is not simply a tool for everyday communication, but through recording of stories, songs, legends, poetry and lore, holds the key to a people's history and opens the door to cultural and spiritual understanding.'[30]

In North America, children of the First Peoples were placed in boarding schools and fostered out and adopted by white mothers. The first boarding school, the Carlisle Institute, was opened in Pennsylvania in 1879 and inspired the federal government to open many more. By 1900, 150 boarding schools and 150 day schools were in operation, containing roughly 21,500 children of the First Peoples.[31] The colonial project of assimilation and extinction via the removal of children was promoted by 'reformers' and discussed as a general strategy by groups who made annual reports, such as Lake Mohonk Conference of the Friends of the Indian and Other Dependent Peoples (1883). Like children in other invaded nations, the American First Peoples children lost their families, language, culture, land, homes and spirituality, a loss that resulted in significant psychological damage to both the abducted children and their grieving communities. There is now abundant evidence that the social and emotional wellbeing of Stolen Generations Survivors and their families is profoundly compromised. The 2004 Western Australian Aboriginal Child Health Survey found that children:

- were 2.3 times more likely to be at high risk of clinically significant emotional or behavioural difficulties after adjusting for age, sex, remoteness and whether the primary carer is the birth mother of the child
- were more likely to be at high risk of clinically significant emotional symptoms, conduct problems and hyperactivity
- had significantly higher rates of overall emotional or behavioural problems in the six months prior to the survey
- had levels of both alcohol and other drug use that were approximately twice as high as children whose Aboriginal primary carer had not been forcibly separated from their natural family.[32]

There is abundant research on the negative impacts of forcibly removing babies and young children from their mothers, institutionalising them, and subjecting them to prolonged psychological, emotional, sexual and physical abuse.[33]

To be clear: *this is a grave human rights issue.*

Such is the ubiquity of this genocidal tactic that the forced removal of First Peoples children can be understood as the disavowed foundation of global colonialism. Many of the early racist policies that sanctioned this fundamental abuse of human rights made it clear, in the manner in which they were written and implemented, that abducting First Peoples children was aimed at extinguishing identity and life itself. In the 2008 Canadian apology offered to the First Peoples for the forced removal of their children, Prime Minister Stephen Harper acknowledged that placing children in 'homes' was done in order 'to kill the Indian in the child'. In this phrase we can hear the distant roar of battle, of an invasion that both legitimised the theft of land as a civilising act and which enforced a genocidal destruction of communities by abducting their children in the name of a civilising rescue mission. Opportunistically framed as children by invading nations, First Peoples are diagnosed as unfit parents, mere children themselves, and their children removed and normalised by a maternal white authority. The phrase 'to kill the Indian in the child' is also the announcement of a broader colonial strategy of indirect killing. In Australia, a colonial myth that the First Peoples were a dying race supported eugenicist policies which were also aimed at destroying communities by removing their children. The Aboriginal Preservation and Protection Act of 1939 recognised the need to protect 'a species which had to be saved from the murderous impulses and practices of settler Australians'.[34] The so-called Protectors, however, targeted children for removal.

The Canadian forced removal of First Peoples children began most intensely in the last few decades of the eighteenth century. Children were removed from their families and communities, placed in Indian Residential Schools, and fostered or adopted by white mothers. As the influential Davin Report of 1879 put it: 'If anything is to be done with the Indian we must catch him very young.'[35] The word 'catch' is significant: children were indeed caught without warning, without consent from their families and communities, a bit like one would catch wild animals. This catching is in effect abduction – an abduction, often violent, that was made in the name of a maternal colonial benevolence but which was saturated with a racist contempt for a people seen as biologically and culturally inferior. As Gwendolyn Point, Education Manager of the Sto:lo (historically written as 'Staulo' or 'Stahlo') Nation in British Columbia, said: 'Ever since the Europeans first came, our children were stolen from our embrace … First the priests took our children away, to churches, schools, even back to Europe. Then the residential schools took three or four generations away.'[36] Moreover, during the 1940s and 1950s starving Indigenous children were subjected to government-run nutritional experiments.

In 1958 a report on Residential Education for Indian Acculturation by Renaud makes clear the project of complex psychological colonisation which drove the removal of children: '[In] acculturating Indian children, the following prescriptions appear necessary for success and thoroughness: isolate the child as much as possible from his native background, ideally twenty four hours a day and twelve months of the year, to prevent "exposure" to Indian culture.'[37] Here acculturation is imagined to be successful to the degree that total separation from culture is achieved. Mothers and fathers, siblings and family are not even mentioned here. Added to this, children 'were subjected to multiple physical, spiritual, sexual, emotional, and cultural abuses'.[38]

Different child-rearing practices

The invading white patriarchal cultures brought with them particular ideologies about children, childhood and the family. The historical construction of whiteness within nations such as Britain is caught up in the policing of childhood by normative discourses about the middle-class family which, far from being child-friendly, expelled children who did not 'fit' (the poor, children of unmarried mothers, Celts, immigrants, Romany and so on) into workhouses, prisons, mines, factories and unmarked graves. Stuffed into the narrow tunnels of mines, worked to the point of death and deformity in textile factories, starved in 'poor houses', prostituted, executed for theft, beaten and murdered with impunity – such was the fate of children who were locked out of the genteel drawing rooms of the British Empire's white middle-class family. The euphemistic term 'baby-farming', for example, described the late eighteenth-century practice of placing the babies of unmarried poor women in 'homes' where many died from deliberate starvation and were buried without recognition. The British parliament recognised the rights of animals before it recognised the rights of children.

As the *Bringing Them Home* report puts it so succinctly:

> In Western terms, welfare as a form of child saving has its origins in late 19th century middle-class concerns about the 'dangerous' classes, single mothers and working-class families in industrialised regions of England.
>
> Many child-savers saw poverty, destitution and the illegal activities of the lower classes as signs of biologically determined character defects. Under the influence of Lombroso, Galtin, Spencer and Darwin, the child-saving movement became a moral crusade, seeking to correct and control the poor ... The [child welfare] system has been predicated on the view that children needed to be rescued from those parents who did not have the innate qualities, right values, correct attitudes and appropriate behaviours considered to be necessary for parents to act in a 'socially acceptable' way.[39]

It is worth recalling, just as the very British cruelty towards children is recalled, that establishing the hegemonic power of the white middle-class patriarchal family over and against First Peoples communities was a key colonial tactic. The white middle-class family was seen as the foundation of all that was good and proper, clean and right, about Western civilisation, while the families of the First Peoples did not really even qualify as families in the eyes of the invading culture. Indeed, it is possible to argue that white supremacism depends on the intimate biological control of the family – children must be bred and brought up in ways that advance the triumph of white civilisation. In this context, the anxieties and aspirations of white supremacism saturate colonial technologies of child-rearing, many of which were inflected with, and provided the grounds for, an emerging discourse of eugenics.

Women's role in the colonial process

In seeking to understand the pattern of global colonial and neocolonial removal of First Peoples children, Jacobs writes in her comparison of the forced removal policies of the Unites States of America and Australia that:

> Although both nations developed similar strategies of removing indigenous children in order to control indigenous populations, there seems to be little evidence of any direct influence of one country upon the other. U.S. officials and reformers did not cite other countries as examples or models for their policy.[40]

Another possible explanation exists. While scholars have yet to trace the network of policy formation between invader nations that spread through the lands of the First Peoples, legitimising the abduction of children, the rise of an international white women's movement during the late nineteenth century is significant insofar as groups such as the World's Woman's Christian Temperance Union, various colonial missionary groups for women, and the Young Women's Christian Association sought to globalise ideals of white middle-class Christian motherhood. The international Suffrage movement also embedded the ideology of white maternalism in colonised lands.[41] Such groups were the result of already existing sociopolitical formations; the discourse of white motherhood, while it might have become an organised event in the late nineteenth century, was still central to the ideological force of colonial white supremacism. 'Ironically, white women maternalists who sought to use their association with motherhood to gain greater power in society were simultaneously engaged in dispossessing indigenous mothers of their children.'[42] White women missionaries, matrons, teachers and nurses were all too often involved in the genocidal wounding of the First Peoples children and communities. Yet white maternalistic interventions into the intimate lives of First Peoples families were promoted as empowering and liberating: numerous self-serving white stories about grateful Indigenous mothers and happy Indigenous children masked the raw reality of child abduction. Stories about the suffering of children and families were carefully silenced.[43]

It was only very rarely that white women spoke out against the removal of children. In a 1937 letter one West Australian woman, Mary Bennett, describes the deliberate starvation of families when voicing her private opposition to the abduction of children:

> [I] implore you NOT to condone or justify taking half-caste children from their aboriginal mothers. The unfortunate mothers are only victims of starvation and to separate parents and children is to destroy both in the most cruel way ... The recent Land Act Amendment of W[estern] A[ustralia] takes away from natives the right to hunt over their tribal lands when these are enclosed, and ... all the native waters are fenced in [by] the [white] squatters ... Their game is destroyed and their dogs are destroyed and the only way they can come by a meal is by selling their women. So I say that W. A. is deliberately starving their natives to death in their own country.'[44]

To starve mothers and then take their children is more than 'cruel' – it is an act of genocide. Bennett prompted a Royal Commission into the oppression of First Peoples in Western Australia. She wrote: 'They are captured at all ages, as infants in arms, perhaps not until they are grown up, *they are not safe until they are dead*' (emphasis added).[45] Perversely, the commission responded by increasing the powers of the white state over all First Peoples:

> Virtually any child of Aboriginal descent could now be taken forcibly from his or her family and placed in a government institution to be trained in the ways of 'white civilisation' and 'society'. The Commissioner of Native Affairs, not their parents, had total control over their lives until they reached the age of twenty-one. From this age any person of 'quarter-caste' or less was prohibited by law from associating with persons deemed to be 'natives'. In this way they were to be forced to live in the white community, although no measures were introduced to force white people to accept them.[46]

Invoking appeals to the superior morality of white parenting, and the correct training of the Christian soul, groups of maternalistic reformers were eager to save 'barbaric' children from their own mothers. 'White women maternalists on both sides of the Pacific justified the "rescue" of indigenous children by focusing on the perceived differences and deficiencies of indigenous women.'[47] Indigenous women were seen as both sexually promiscuous and as the victims of a brutally barbaric male-dominated culture. They were also seen as unfit mothers who did not understand the very basics of child rearing, to the point where it was assumed they did not even know how to carry their children 'correctly' or provide them with safe homes, and who were continually placing their children in physical, emotional, psychological, sexual and spiritual danger.[48] Jacobs writes that 'while maternalist ideologies and politics potentially empowered white middle-class Protestant women, they served to further colonial aims by eroding indigenous women's authority within their own societies'.[49]

A generalised white moral panic about the sexual depravity of Indigenous men was also a central narrative. 'Many white women reformers believed it was essential to remove indigenous children, particularly girls, from their families to protect them from what white women perceived to be sexual exploitation and abuse.'[50] Significantly, this colonial moral panic about Indigenous child sexual abuse is a resilient racist narrative, one that continues to legitimise the removal of children from families. The racist stereotype of the sexually depraved black man, who is so lacking in sexual boundaries that he abuses children, supported the passing of the Northern Territory National Emergency

Response Act of 2007, which led to the 2007 Northern Territory Emergency Response. This event reanimated centuries-old racist beliefs about the primitive sexuality of First Peoples men. As though forced to carry a white man's projection and become the shadow of the sexual exploitation of women and children by white invaders, First Peoples men are demonised and insulted, just as their ability to protect their children is overwhelmed by colonial violence. As Mick Adams writes:

> Aboriginal and Torres Strait Islander men have been disempowered through the reduction of their authority and status, and also because of restrictions on their cultural activities and values … Aboriginal and Torres Strait Islander men have been displaced and are still subjected to abuse, marginalisation and racism within the wider Australian society.[51]

Many of these men were also stolen from their families as children, and abused and exploited as children by hostile whites.

Although the discourses that compose the sociopolitical laboratory of colonialism and neocolonialism are numerous, complex and contradictory, the idea that Indigenous people are childlike and, in the case of the First Peoples of Australia, at the bottom of the Darwinian evolutionary hierarchy, the most childish, the most lacking, is a dominant narrative which is still deployed against Indigenous people. The maternalistic racism directed at First Peoples by invading nations, this peering down at, head patting and enforcing of disciplinary policies which are made 'for their own good', is intimately entwined with Western child-rearing discourses. Such discourses, with their Western ideas of normal and abnormal development, provided multiple excuses for breaking and remaking children, families and communities. Colonial maternalism is also opportunistic insofar as the economic motive behind the framing of Indigenous people as childlike primitives, namely the theft of land and the exploitation of its people, is masked by a rhetoric of motherly benevolence. In Australia the white state even named itself 'Protectors' as it continued to take land and children. By 1911 all states in Australia implemented legislation for removing Indigenous children from their parents and communities.

As it is now well documented, the surviving Stolen Generations have the highest suicide rates, score lowest in social and emotional wellbeing, are incarcerated more frequently and have children and grandchildren who are also impacted.[52] The psychological impact on families and communities who have had their children removed is also another form of wounding. It is as though 'killing the Indian in the child' was a normative technology that was then transmitted through the bodies of members of Stolen Generations, as though the spiritual and psychological murder spreads outwards, so that it is not just the 'Indian in the child' that is killed but the Indian in the mother, father, brother, sister, aunt, uncle, grandmother, grandfather, friend – the community.

The Stolen Generations of First Peoples children in Australia

> The authorities forcibly took her child, Lillian, in 1909 to be assimilated and civilised. I have thought about how it may have happened – did Bella run screaming and wailing after the party that took her 11-year-old daughter away? Was she stopped dead in her terror-filled flight to save her child, and then beaten down into the red dust? Her sisters would have gathered around her, protecting, wailing and grieving. Did she grieve and beat her head with sharp stones as they did when a loved one died, the physical pain and blood an expression of the heart's anguish? The state and the church thought that Aboriginal women would quickly get over the removal of their children (Choo, 2001), like bitch dogs who have their litters taken. The tragedy of colonisation for Bella at a very personal level is that, as well as making Aboriginal people less than human, they also dehumanised and devalued her mother's love.[53]
>
> My mother had to come with us. She had already lost her eldest daughter down to the Children's Hospital because she had infantile paralysis, polio, and now there was the prospect of losing her three other children, all the children she had. I remember that she came in the truck with us curled up in the foetal position. Who can understand that, the trauma of knowing that you're going to lose all your children? We talk about it from the point of view of our trauma but – our mother – to understand what she went through, I don't think anyone can really understand that.[54]
>
> (Pat Dudgeon, reflecting in 2008 and 2015 on her foremothers' experience of removal).

In 1997 the Australian Human Rights and Equal Opportunity Commission released the lengthy and rigorously researched *Bringing Them Home: Report of the National Inquiry into the Separation of Aboriginal and Torres Strait Islander Children from their Families* after the Attorney-General of Australia, Michael Levarch, commissioned an inquiry in 1995 under the government of Paul Keating. The report argued, *thoroughly*, that Australia had breached British common law and international law, in particular the United Nations Convention Against Genocide, in its treatment of First Peoples children and their families. The report details generations of systematic child sexual abuse and neglect inflicted, with impunity, on First Peoples children by white people. Eleven years after the *Bringing Them Home* report the neocolonial Australian government responded with a carefully worded apology to the Stolen Generations. Moreover, although the *Bringing Them Home* report had called for reparation for First Peoples, the ruling white government made it clear 11 years later that this would not occur. Some 16 years after the government apology, reparation is still refused. Indeed, in 2014 a former Prime Minister of Australia, John Howard, publicly stated that the *Bringing Them Home* report was false and (once again) denied the genocide of First Peoples.[55]

'Indigenous children have been forcibly separated from their families and communities since the very first days of the European occupation of Australia.'[56] These early child abductions had a clear economic motive: quite simply, white settlers exploited First Peoples children as slaves.[57] The first white enclosure for First Peoples children, the Native Institution in Parramatta, was opened in 1814 by Governor Macquarie. Resistance from families resulted in closure in 1820, but many other institutions were created. In the Australian state of Victoria between 1838 and 1849, government-appointed 'Protectors of Aborigines' intensified the removal of children from 'tribal influences' and, as was often the case, once the children were taken they were declared 'orphans'.[58] By 1890 the infamous Aborigines Protection Board responded to the growing numbers of children with white biological fathers by seeking to forcibly remove them from their mothers and families. By 1893 a girls' dormitory was built at Warangesda Station, which housed 300 children between 1893 and 1909.

In 1909 the Aborigines Protection Act legislated the ability of the colonial government to 'assume full control and custody of the child of any Aborigine' if children were found to be neglected under the 1905 Neglected Children and Juvenile Offenders Act. Idealised myths of the white middle-class family influenced definitions of neglect, inevitably framing First Peoples communities as abusive. Moreover, impoverished parents were at a great disadvantage in white courts, which used a combative and foreign language. By 1915 the Aborigines Protection Amending Act did away with the need to prove neglect in the courts. 'Apart from just "being Aboriginal" other commonly cited reasons for removal were "To send to service", "Being 14 years", "At risk of immorality",

"Neglected", "To get her away from surroundings of Aboriginal station/ Removal from idle reserve life" and "Orphan".'[59] Significantly, the 1915 amendment 'abolished the minimum age at which Aboriginal children could be apprenticed'.[60] It is reasonable then, to deduce that the forced removal of children may have had another underlying agenda in the exploitation of child labour by whites. In 1913 a Royal Commission was established 'to inquire into and report upon the control, organisation and management of institutions ... set aside for the benefit of Aborigines'. Various white male officials discussed the best age for removing children from their mothers. 'The Secretary of the State Children's Council argued that they should be taken away as infants. "If they are in the wurley [a name for a First Peoples' shelter] for a week it is bad for them, but it is fatal for them to remain there a year."'[61] Others disagreed:

> Professor Stirling from the University of Adelaide, on the other hand, argued that the best time to take Aboriginal children was when they were about two years old.
>
> 'The more of those half-caste children you can take away from their parents and place under the care of the State the better ... When they are a couple of years of age they do not require so much attention and they are young enough to be attractive.'
>
> I am quite aware that you are depriving the mothers of their children, and the mothers are very fond of their children; but I think it must be the rising generation who have to be considered. They are the people who are going to live on.[62]

Misgivings are raised about the comment 'young enough to be attractive'. To whom and why should a child be attractive? One hopes that it might refer to the 'unspoiled' appearance and nature of the child – like a puppy or a kitten – that led to this unfortunate comment.

During the height of the eugenics movement in the 1920s and 1930s vast numbers of children were removed. By 1921, 81 per cent of the recorded children removed were girls, and girls continued to be disproportionately represented by 1939.[63] Significant numbers of boys were imprisoned.

The relentless criminal assault against First Peoples through government acts steadily degraded communities. In Western Australia the 1947 Child Welfare Act was used against First Peoples communities. In 1954 the Native Welfare Act resulted in the Commissioner for Native Affairs being the legal guardian of all First Peoples children except those who were already wards of the white state, a guardianship that only changed with the passing of the Native Welfare Act of 1963. In 1965 the Adoption of Children Act gave further powers of removal by once again deploying culturally inappropriate concepts of child neglect.[64] The ominously titled Chief Protectors and associated white officials were the legal guardians of all First Peoples children until 1963 in Western Australia, 1964 in the Northern Territory, 1962 in South Australia and 1965 in Queensland.[65] As the *Bringing Them Home* report states: 'Nationally we can conclude with confidence that between one in three and one in ten Indigenous children were forcibly removed from their families and communities in the period from approximately 1910 until 1970.'[66]

The degree of abuse and neglect reported is, quite simply, horrific, and to read the full report and the numerous atrocities committed is a traumatic experience in itself. It is clear that the systemic government- and Church-sanctioned abuse of children by whites constitutes a serious crime against humanity. In short, not only were children forcibly removed from their families; they were all too often subjected to severe maltreatment, physical and sexual abuse, gross humiliation, starvation and severely reduced living conditions, and sustained psychological abuse which was often extremely racist; they were separated from siblings, lied to about their parents and family, shuttled from one abusive foster home to another, actively prevented from making contact with their family, and, in some cases, tortured and murdered. There are also details of generations of parents suffering nervous breakdowns and dying from the trauma of having their children forcibly removed by a hostile and racist authoritarian system which had already persecuted them in their own country.

Resistance

Resistance by First Peoples against the abduction of children was and is continuous, but this history is only now emerging. Many women resistance leaders had, and continue to have, key roles in combatting child abduction by the white Australian government. Jane Duren, for example, in the first national Indigenous political body, the Australian Aboriginal Progressive Association (AAPA) (which was headed by Charles Maynard in 1924) targeted the New South Wales Aboriginal Protection Board which forcibly removed children from their mothers. Writing to the Premier in 1927 Maynard suggested 'that the family life of Aboriginal people shall be held sacred and free from invasion and interference and that the children shall be left in the control of their parents'.[67] During the intense wave of civil rights action in the 1960s and 1970s, and with the brief support of the Whitlam government, the removal of children was challenged by newly created First Peoples legal services and the Victorian Aboriginal and Islander Child Care Agency (AICCA), the first of its kind.[68] Australian Adoption Conferences in 1976, 1978 and 1982 highlighted for the first time the grievous impact of forced removals. The Aboriginal Children's Services was established in New South Wales in 1975. The First Aboriginal Child Survival Conference was held in 1979.[69] Molly Dyer, the daughter of Margaret Tucker, was successful in creating the Aboriginal Child Placement Principle, which recognised that removed Aboriginal children should be placed with Aboriginal families. This successful policy was rolled out by many welfare departments in the 1980s.[70] Significantly, in 1980 the first Link-Up Aboriginal Corporation devoted to researching and reuniting families was formed in New South Wales. The 1997 *Bringing Them Home* report detailed how in '1981 the Secretariat of National Aboriginal and Islander Child Care (SNAICC) was formed and there are now approximately 100 Aboriginal community-run children's services under its umbrella'.[71]

Barbara Cummings, a victim of forced removal as a child, documented the forced removal of children in the Northern Territory in her authoritative 1990 book *Take this Child: From Kahlin Compound to Retta Dixon Children's Home*. She organised the 1996 Going Home Conference in Darwin after the 1995 start of the National Inquiry into the Separation of Aboriginal and Torres Strait Islander Children from their Families, and with other women created the Karu Aboriginal Family Support Agency and the Aboriginal and Islander Child Care Agency in Darwin.[72] In 2014 the New South Wales Gunnedah grandmothers formed to challenge the continuing removal of children from their mothers by various state governments. In 2015 the energetic resurgence of a First Peoples civil rights movement is highlighting the continuing removal of children as a central issue.

First People healing: communal parenting

Broadly speaking, the Australian Indigenous mental health movement is building resistance against the complex trauma of neocolonialism both by decolonising child-rearing practices through the restoration of culturally appropriate child-rearing in communities, and by developing community-based healing practices that address the genocidal wounding caused by generations of forced removals of children. Very broadly,

Indigenous child-rearing and healing is a communal process. Despite concerted efforts by the invading culture to discipline and control Indigenous people within the alienating structures of the white nuclear family, communal parenting and healing continues.

Before invasion, diversely and intricately structured families and communities were raising happy and healthy children, passing on an oral culture through parenting and other attachment relationships. The communal bonds between children, parents and the whole community were and are integral to the development of a healthy identity and the ability to form relationships with others. This process is governed by internal working models which are exercised and refined in the parenting relationship. Such relations are unequivocally driven by cultural values, defining what 'should' be a good parenting model, detailing the various scripts for raising children, including how to feed, bathe, discipline and teach social skills.[73] In contrast to the Western nuclear family, Indigenous parenting is a collective process – by imposing the foreign individualistic culture on Aboriginal and Torres Strait Islander peoples, the collective working models and cultural scripts for raising children were disrupted and destroyed. Moreover, colonisation did more than just disrupt the developmental foundations of identity; colonisation took away the material and spiritual foundation within which such development was formed – the land itself. As a consequence, the foundations of intimacy within communities were damaged. Evidence for this damage is widely documented in the poor health and wellbeing of Aboriginal adults and social, emotional and behavioural problems in children.

There have been widely documented differences between individualistic and collectivist societies. Individualistic cultures value the individual before the community while collectivist society members align their values with those of the community. This affects the way parenting knowledge and values are transmitted through the generations. Keller proposed that different parenting strategies across cultures are related to different developmental goals and that this is connected to whether the culture is individualistic or collectivist.[74] This poses a problem for an individualistic Western society imposing their parenting style on a more collectivist Aboriginal style of parenting.

The transmission of parenting strategies is through these internal working models. The detailed scripts would be built upon individualistic values or collectivist values, directing parenting behaviours to support the developmental goals of the culture. When the collectivist Aboriginal and Torres Strait Islander culture was physically invaded by the English individualistic culture, so too was the psychological and spiritual realm of Aboriginal people. The physical result of the clash of cultures has been masking the internal psychological damage of the invasion. High rates of suicide, illness and death due to oppression, incarceration and self-medication with drugs and alcohol physically takes parents away from their children while the interference of culture – internal working models – takes parents away on a psychological level. This leaves children growing up with a potentially unsafe physical environment and an equally unsafe internal environment.

Present-day realities for Aboriginal families include governmental policies designed to keep Aboriginal families apart because of a mistrust of their parenting abilities, and forced displacement from traditional lands for economic reasons, ultimately resulting in separation from family and kinship systems.[75] Trauma is suffered from being removed, and fresh trauma results from the new environment. In this way, the trauma of neocolonialism is compounded and intensified.

In short, government policies of assimilation destroy attachment bonds between children and parents, families and community. Forced removals also cause post-traumatic symptoms for both children and parents, which impair the ability to nurture the self and others. Traumatised and deprived of healthy attachment bonds, Indigenous parents then struggle to raise childen who can view themselves lovingly. Forced separation leaves children with a poor self-concept and traumatised internal working models. These children then grow into adults who have no experience of being parented themselves, or they experience inconsistent parenting, with varying levels of care and control dependent on where they were placed, leaving their internal working models pieced together with information from whatever they were exposed to, be it good or bad. Generations of these children grow into parents who are poorly internally organised and poorly equipped to raise children. Moreover, persistent racist discrimination against First Peoples children, mothers, fathers and whole communities in neocolonial Australia; lack of adequate housing; educational and employment disadvantage; not to mention the ongoing trauma of genocide all mean that the bonds between children and parents are being undermined by the dominant white culture.

However, despite this destruction, Aboriginal and Torres Strait Islander people have been incredibly resilient. The resilience of Aboriginal and Torres Strait Islander people is just beginning to be documented in research across many disciplines. Although empirical research has yet to be documented on Indigenous parenting, early anecdotal evidence points to a communal style of raising children, with the parental responsibilities shared amongst extended family members.[76] This reflection of traditional ways indicates that First Peoples communities have resisted individualistic, white, nuclear-family-style parenting. Contact with people and land may have been sustaining enough to continue with some adherence to traditional parenting practices.

Several protective factors generated by the community itself have been identified in studies of First Peoples families. These include a strong family system and role models, quality child care, parents monitoring children's health status, feelings of connectedness between child and parent, access to culturally appropriate healthcare, opportunities for learning about culture and socialising (through sporting and culturally supported activities), and community support networks outside the immediate family. Aboriginal parents studied in *Footprints in Time – The Longitudinal Study of Indigenous Children* believe that children can benefit from playing sport, having goals and receiving a good education, and that looking after children with the support of extended family raises kids that can look after themselves.[77] They believe it is the parents' job to encourage resilience in children: putting their identity as a priority, maintaining a strong family influence, teaching children how to deal with racism in a mature way, teaching them the power of being alive and the meaning of being Aboriginal, and alerting children to the danger of drug addicts and child abusers.

The lack of empirical evidence about Indigenous parenting means that current policy is written on anecdotal evidence which may not be accurate. Two recent studies have attempted to capture the nature of Indigenous parenting. The authors collected family stories concerning child-rearing, development, behaviour, health and wellbeing of 15 infants from birth to their first birthday. They found significant differences in parenting behaviours and child-rearing practices between Aboriginal groups and 'mainstream' Australians. Aboriginal parents perceived their children to be autonomous individuals with responsibilities towards the community, and the children were active agents in determining their own needs.[78]

The study found that relationship-building began at birth with lots of communication to the baby about their place in the community and lots of affection from family and community members. At this young age the father and other family members were responsible for supporting the mother so she could care for her child. As the child grew older the collective stepped in and took several child-rearing roles in the child's life.

In terms of behaviour control, caregivers created fear in children or distracted them rather than saying 'No don't do this'. This indirect approach to behaviour control reinforced the notion that children are autonomous individuals and active decision-makers. Family members were never punitive to their children and didn't judge them, although they did describe them as being cheeky. The mothers did not enforce routines on their babies and instead were responsive to their babies' needs. This supported the observation that the families responded to the infants' specific needs, providing care on an individual, child-led basis.

An important finding in this study was the Aboriginal belief that each child is an independent autonomous human being capable of communicating and determining his or her needs from birth, and that the entire family group is responsible for responding to those needs. Failure to do so is considered cruel and damaging to the infant's wellbeing and autonomy. Researchers have found similar parenting characteristics which situate the child as the active agent in determining his or her needs from birth.[79]

The findings of this study do not support the allocation of this group of Aboriginal parents to any of the known Western parenting categories. For example, Aboriginal parents' awareness of the child's level of development in relation to peer groups does not assume the same importance as it does for families dominated by discourses of white mainstream developmental milestones.[80] This absence of self-surveillance suggests that Aboriginal families are not controlled by the normalising regimes of Western child development discourses.

This study is in line with a descriptive study that was carried out in a remote central Australian community working with eight families with children under five.[81] Data were collected through participant observation and informal conversation interviews. Three main interlinked themes were identified through the research: the integration of children into community life, differing views of children's development, and encouraging children's autonomy within a communal social structure. In this community the development of independence and self-reliance within a closely nurturing environment were the most important parenting tasks. Children were taught responsibilities and social obligations through interaction and community life from birth. Fathers were tasked with the job of skilling up children to fit in with their peers while mothers and others educated children using verbal warnings and modelling of social norms. Children were taught socially appropriate behaviour through being shamed, and teasing was used to distract children from something 'naughty' they were doing, which is vastly different from non-Aboriginal parenting. Shaming is not included in non-Aboriginal parenting behaviour-management strategies.[82]

Nelson and Allison have identified an alternative Indigenous parenting style termed 'intuitive'.[83] These parents intuitively encourage their child's learning and development from birth but the specific knowledge and skills taught may vary amongst Aboriginal subcultures. It is thought that this Indigenous parenting style will result in children with a high sense of personal competence. In their qualitative study of Aboriginal parental values, participants described six parental values: survival, safety, social relationships, esteem (achieving and leadership), cognitive needs and self-actualisation. The aim of this parenting strategy was to maintain social harmony while ensuring the safety of the children.

These studies illustrate the resilience not only of Indigenous people but of Indigenous families and parenting. The collectivist values filtering through the parenting strategies are evident in the *Footprints in Time* survey of Indigenous parenting, connecting to family, community and culture from birth.

The lessons learnt from this research filter outwards from the family, through community and to society. Imposing Western perspectives on Aboriginal knowledge contributes to three problems: first, Aboriginal families are at risk of being misunderstood by service providers and governmental departments that may be making decisions about their family members; second, important information that could contribute to the positive development of Aboriginal children tends to be 'lost' owing to the lack of empirical research; and third, imposing any other model of child-rearing on Aboriginal parents devalues the validity of other ways of 'knowing' and reinforces discrimination.[84] 'Hence, until the planners of Australia's health systems better understand Aboriginal knowledge systems and incorporate them into their planning, we can continue to expect the failure of government and health services among Aboriginal communities.'[85] First Peoples families must also contend with the emotional, spiritual, psychological and socioeconomic trauma of colonisation.

Healing incalculable trauma

Genocidal colonisation is a process of complex and chronic dehumanising trauma. As Atkinson et al argue, the complexity of the trauma exceeds classical (Western) definitions of post-traumatic stress disorder (PTSD) precisely because the stress experienced by Indigenous Australians is severe, persistent, culminative, multiple, and inflicted by a hostile and dominant authoritarian white culture. In recognition of this complex form of trauma the Australian Aboriginal Version of the Harvard Trauma Questionnaire (AAVHTQ) was developed by Atkinson in order to provide a culturally competent measurement of particular traumatic stressors and symptoms.[86] Atkinson identifies the forced removal of children as a significant source of trauma, not only because it is in itself traumatic for any child and mother to be forcibly separated, but also because this abduction occurs within the context of *ongoing genocide*. Moreover, as Peeters, Hamann and Kelly point out, the complex and continuous human rights abuses experienced by people forcibly removed as children and then exploited and abused cannot be contained by the pathologising label of post-traumatic stress disorder. 'PTSD participates in a process that converts a social and political problem into psychopathology. "D" stands for disorder. There is probably nothing less helpful for a victim of human rights violations than to classify his or her suffering as a mental illness.'[87]

The Sydney Aboriginal Mental Health Unit, which advised the *Bringing Them Home* inquiry of its experience with patients presenting with emotional distress, described the extent of the trauma as 'incalculable':

> This tragic experience, across several generations, has resulted in incalculable trauma, depression and major mental health problems for Aboriginal people. Careful history taking during the assessment of most individuals (i.e. clients) and families identifies separation by one means or another – initially the systematic removal of children … has been tantamount to a continuing cultural and spiritual genocide both as an individual and a community experience and we believe that it has been the single most significant factor in emotional and mental health problems which in turn have impacted on physical health.[88]

In response to this severe damage, Indigenous psychology has emerged as a powerful force for healing within communities and has led the way in establishing numerous programs which seek to re-empower First Peoples. As Dudgeon, Walker et al state:

> When considering the impacts of trauma experienced historically, there are three major themes that cover the nature of the trauma that occurred over many generations and continue to be experienced. These are:

- the extreme sense of powerlessness and loss of control;
- the profound sense of loss, grief and disconnection; and
- the overwhelming sense of trauma and helplessness.

In turn, there are three pathways to recovery to address each of these areas of trauma that have occurred as a consequence of the history of colonisation and its impacts:

- self-determination and community governance;
- reconnection and community life; and
- restoration and community resilience.

Most significantly we argue that an Aboriginal worldview, developing a comprehensive, holistic approach that focuses on individual, family and community strengths whilst at the same time addressing the needs of the community, is both a more culturally acceptable and effective approach to address these issues.[89]

Of particular concern is the epidemic of youth suicide within First Peoples communities, which is one of the highest in the world. Healing Aboriginal social and emotional wellbeing is beyond the capabilities of Western mental health programmes which risk imposing traumatic interventions on already traumatised communities.

Of significance is the National Empowerment Program, led by Dudgeon, which has identified the need for further programmes that build on and recognise the innate strength and resilience of First Peoples and implement culturally wise empowerment.[90] The Hear Our Voices project, also led by Dudgeon, consulted many communities and 'highlighted the importance of listening to Aboriginal people who themselves identified healing, empowerment and leadership as three critical elements in meeting their needs and aspirations'.[91] Aunty Lorraine Peeters has created the significant Marumali Journey of Healing programmes which address the unique trauma facing survivors of forced removal. 'For us, healing involves mind, body, spirit, spirituality, family, culture and sometimes (if we are lucky) country,' she says. 'It is about finding our "belonging place", whatever that might mean to each of us.'[92] Voices from the Campfire (2009), a national consultation undertaken by the Aboriginal and Torres Strait Islander Healing Foundation, 'found that Aboriginal participants saw healing as a spiritual journey that requires initiatives to assist in the recovery from trauma and addiction, and reconnection to the family, community and culture'.[93] A key finding in many consultations and programmes is that healing is a whole-community event and that merely focusing on a (pathologised) individual, as the Western style of approach most typically does, achieves very little. Suicide prevention and the restoration of social and emotional wellbeing are, logically, a dynamic process which holds the whole of the community. Moreover, focusing on traumatic wounding as a community issue avoids the ahistorical, decontextual and, indeed, apolitical approach which dominates Western psychology, and empowers people to acknowledge the impact of colonialism rather than blaming individuals within communities. In this way, collective social change is built from the ground up. A key feature of these programmes is a recognition that health is a holistic practice which respects the intimate 'interconnectedness of life's dimension'.[94] In this context, all that has been stolen from First Peoples – land, spirituality, language, family, home, health, life, security, love itself – is recovered and reconnected with.

Conclusion: self-determination

The challenges facing the First Peoples of Australia are significant. Genocidal practices have not ceased and racism towards First Peoples, of all ages, regardless of sex or class, continues to harm in overt and covert ways. This chapter has drawn attention to a principle cause of deep suffering for First Peoples – generations of forced removal of children – within the context of a neocolonial culture that still perpetrates racism. The strength of First Peoples' resistance can be witnessed in the recent rise of national healing movements which are based on the principles of self-determination.

The first step in re-establishing healthy communities is to acknowledge and understand the impact of the colonial legacy on the lives of Aboriginal people today and the various pathways necessary for healing from historical trauma, using both cultural and contemporary understandings and processes. Although the full history of Australia in regard to the treatment of Aboriginal peoples remains in dispute, there is enough evidence to support the experience of sustained, profound trauma for the entire Aboriginal community over generations, suggestive of *genocide*.

It is partly the ongoing effects of this process, which continue to impact negatively at the individual and community level, that require healing, before the contemporary issues can be successfully dealt with. Following this, establishing appropriate cultural, community, family and individual support systems and programmes, to address current needs and developments, can occur systematically.

Take a moment to stop and think about this. What if this had happened to you or your children? How would you feel now? [95]

Endnotes

1. National Inquiry into the Separation of Aboriginal and Torres Strait Islander Children from Their Families (1997). *Bringing Them Home: Report of the national inquiry into the separation of Aboriginal and Torres Strait Islander children from their families.* Sydney: Human Rights and Equal Opportunity Commission, Commonwealth of Australia, p. 6.
2. Mills, S. (2014). 'I am sorry': Prime ministerial apology as transformational leadership. In J. Uhr & R. Walter (Eds) *Studies in Australian Political Rhetoric* (pp. 19–32). Canberra: Australian National University Press, p. 22.
3. Georgatos, G. (2015). Highest child removal rates in the world — worse than Stolen Generations. *The Stringer*, 15 February 2015. Available at http://thestringer.com.au/highest-child-removal-rates-in-the-world-worse-than-stolen-generations-9554#.VWKfrlYWeqQ (retrieved 25 May 2015).
4. Sinclair, R. (2007). Lost and found: Lessons from the sixties scoop. *First Peoples Child and Family Review: A journal on innovation and best practice in Aboriginal child welfare administration, research, policy and practice, 3* (1) 65–82; de Finney, S., Dean, M., Loiselle, E. & Saraceno, J. (2011). All children are equal, but some are more equal than others: Minoritization, structural inequities, and social justice praxis in residential care. *International Journal of Child, Youth and Family Studies, 3 & 4,* 361–384, p. 369.
5. Dudgeon, P., Milroy, H. & Walker, R. (Eds) (2014). *Working Together: Aboriginal and Torres Strait Islander mental health and wellbeing principles and practice* (2nd edition). Canberra: Commonwealth of Australia.
6. Haebich, A. (2000). *Broken Circles.* Fremantle: Fremantle Arts Centre Press, p. 13.
7. *Bringing Them Home,* 1997, p. 31. See note 1.
8. McGrath, 1995, p. 93. See note 17.
9. Haebich, 2000, p. 13. See note 6.
10. Dudgeon, P. & Walker, R. (2015). Decolonizing Australian psychology: Discourses, strategies and practices. *Journal of Social and Political Psychology.* (In press).
11. Tuhiwai Smith, L. (1999). *Decolonizing Methodologies: Research and indigenous peoples.* London: Zed Books.
12. Moreton-Robinson, A. M. (2003). I still call Australia home: Indigenous belonging and place in a white postcolonising society. In S. Ahmed (Ed.). *Uprootings/Regroundings: Questions of home and migration* (pp. 23–40). Oxford: Berg, p. 30.
13. Anderson, I. (1995). Re-Claiming TRU-GER-NAN-NER: Decolonising the symbol. In P. van Toorn & D. English (Eds). *Speaking Positions: Aboriginality, gender and ethnicity in Australian cultural studies* (pp. 31–42). Melbourne: Victoria University of Technology, p. 38.
14. Moreton-Robinson, A. M. (2003). I still call Australia home: Indigenous belonging and place in a white postcolonising society. In S. Ahmed (Ed.). *Uprootings/Regroundings: Questions of home and migration* (pp. 23–40). Oxford: Berg, p. 30.

15. Bhabha, H. (2008). Forward to the 1986 edition. In F. Fanon, *Black Skin, White Masks* (trans. Lam Markmann). London: Pluto Press, pp. xxi–xxxvii.
16. Dudgeon, P. & Bray, A. (2014). Disabling the First People: Re-scientized racism and the Indigenous mental health movement. *The Journal of Critical Psychology, Counselling and Psychotherapy, 14* (4) 226–237.
17. McGrath, A. (1995). *Contested Ground: Australian Aborigines under the British Crown*. Sydney: Allen & Unwin.
18. Ibid. p. 1.
19. Broome, R. (1994). *Aboriginal Australians: Black responses to white dominance, 1788–1994* (2nd edition). Sydney: Allen & Unwin.
20. McGrath, 1995. See note 17.
21. Stanner, W. E. H. (1969). *After the Dreaming: Black and white Australians – an anthropologist's view*. Sydney: Australian Broadcasting Commission; Stanner, W. E. H. (1969). *The Boyer Lectures 1968 – After the Dreaming*. Sydney: Australian Broadcasting Commission.
22. Rowley, C. D. (1970). *The Destruction of Aboriginal Society*. Canberra: The Australian National University Press; Rowley, C. D. (1971a). *The Remote Aborigines*. Canberra: The Australian National University Press; Rowley, C. D. (1971b). *Outcasts in White Australia*. Canberra: The Australian National University Press; Rowley, C. D. (1986). *Recovery: The politics of Aboriginal reform*. Canberra: The Australian National University Press; Reynolds, H. (1999). *Why Weren't We Told?* Ringwood, Victoria: Penguin; Broome, R. (1982). *Aboriginal Australians: Black response to white dominance, 1788–1980*. Sydney: George Allen and Unwin; Biskup, P. (1973). *Not Slaves, Not Citizens: The Aboriginal problem in Western Australia 1898–1954*. Sydney: Taylor and Francis.
23. Moreton-Robinson, 2003, p. 128. See note 14.
24. Tuhiwai Smith, L. (1999). *Decolonizing Methodologies: Research and indigenous peoples*. London: Zed Books.
25. Morgan, S. (2002). *Echoes of the Past: Sister Kate's home revisited*. Perth: Centre for Indigenous History and the Arts, University of Western Australia.
26. Sissons, J. (2005). *First Peoples: Indigenous cultures and their futures*. Chicago: University of Chicago press.
27. Bull, S. & Alia, V. (2004). Unequaled acts of injustice: Pan-indigenous encounters with colonial school systems. *Contemporary Justice Review: Issues in criminal, social, and restorative justice, 7* (2) 171–182, p. 176.
28. Haig-Brown, C. (1988). *Resistance and Renewal: Surviving the Indian residential school*. Vancouver: Arsenal Pulp Press, p. 16.
29. Ibid. p. 15.
30. *Bringing Them Home*, 1997, p. 259. See note 1.
31. Jacobs, M. D. (2005). Maternal Colonialism: White women and indigenous child removal in the American West and Australia, 1880–1940 [online]. Lincoln, NE: University of Nebraska Department of History. Available at http://digitalcommons.unl.edu/historyfacpub/11 (retrieved 3 May 2015), p. 459.
32. Australian Bureau of Statistics (2010). *The Health and Welfare of Australia's Aboriginal and Torres Strait Islander Peoples*. Available at http://www.abs.gov.au/ausstats/abs@.nsf/mf/4704.0 (retrieved 8 June 2015).
33. *Bringing Them Home*, 1997, pp. 158–174. See note 1.
34. Tatz, C. (1999). Genocide in Australia. *Journal of Genocide Research, 1* (3) 315–352, p. 316.
35. Davin, N. F. (1879). *Report on Industrial Schools for Indians and Half-breeds*. Report presented to the Government of Canada, Ottawa, p. 2.
36. Quoted in Fournier, S. & Crey, E. (1997). *Stolen From Our Embrace: The abduction*

of First Nations children and the restoration of aboriginal communities. Vancouver: Douglas & McIntyre, pp. 7–8.
37. Renaud, A., (1958). Indian education today. *Anthropologica*, 6, 1–49, p. 34.
38. de Finney, S., Dean, M., Loiselle, E. & Saraceno, J. (2011). All children are equal, but some are more equal than others: Minoritization, structural inequities, and social justice praxis in residential care. *International Journal of Child, Youth and Family Studies*, 3 & 4, 361–384, p. 369.
39. *Bringing Them Home*, 1997, pp. 375–376. See note 1.
40. Jacobs, 2005, pp. 459–560. See note 31.
41. Ibid. pp. 465–466.
42. Ibid. p. 476.
43. Ibid. p. 469.
44. Mary Bennett to Olive Pink, 12 September 1937, I. F. (a) (2), *Olive Pink Papers*, Australian Institute for Aboriginal and Torres Strait Islander Studies, Canberra.
45. *Bringing Them Home*, 1997, p. 94. See note 1.
46. Haebich, 2000, p. 351. See note 6.
47. Jacobs, 2005, p. 462. See note 31.
48. Kearins, J. (1991). Visual spatial memory in Aboriginal and white Australian children. In K. M. McConkey & N. W. Bonds (Eds). *Readings in Australian Psychology* (pp. 197–208). Sydney: Harcourt Brace, Jovanovich.
49. Jacobs, 2005, p. 465. See note 31.
50. Ibid. p. 463.
51. Adams, M. (n.d.). Working towards changing the negative image of Aboriginal and Torres Strait Islander males [unpublished manuscript]. Fineline Consultancy.
52. Skott-Myhre, H. (2005). Towards a minoritarian psychology of immanence and a psychotherapy of flight: Political meditations on the society of control. *Parallax*, 11 (2) 44–59.
53. Peeters, L., Hamann, S. & Kelly, K. (2014). The Marumali program: Healing for stolen generations. In P. Dudgeon, H. Milroy & R. Walker (Eds). *Working Together: Aboriginal and Torres Strait Islander mental health and wellbeing principles and practice* (2nd edition) (pp. 493–507). Canberra: Commonwealth of Australia.
54. Dudgeon, P. (In press). Mothers of sin: Indigenous women's perceptions of their identity and sexuality/gender. In P. Dudgeon, H. Milroy, D. Oxenham & A. Herbert (Eds). *Our Women, Our Ways*. Broome: Magabala Books; Choo, C. (2001). *Mission Girls: Aboriginal women on Catholic missions in the Kimberley, Western Australia, 1900–1950*. Perth: University of Western Australia Press.
55. Davidson, H. (2014). 'There is no genocide against Indigenous Australians': Former PM says he did not accept the conclusion of the Bringing Them Home Report. *The Guardian*, 22 September. Available at http://www.theguardian.com/world/2014/sep/22/john-howard-there-was-no-genocide-against-indigenous-australians (retrieved 25 May 2015).
56. *Bringing Them Home*, 1997, p. 111. See note 1.
57. Ibid. p. 22.
58. Reynolds, H. (1990). *With the White People: The crucial role of Aborigines in the exploration and development of Australia*. Ringwood, Victoria: Penguin Books, p. 169. See also Peeters, L., Hamann, S. & Kelly, K. (2014). The Marumali program: Healing for stolen generations. In P. Dudgeon, H. Milroy & R. Walker (Eds). *Working Together: Aboriginal and Torres Strait Islander mental health and wellbeing principles and practice* (2nd edition) (pp. 493–507). Canberra: Commonwealth of Australia; and Sovereign Union (n.d.). First Australians: Historic resources and activism links [online].

Available at http://www.nationalunitygovernment.org/content/first-australians-historic-resources-and-activism-links (retrieved 3 May 2015).
59. *Bringing Them Home*, 1997, p. 50. See note 1.
60. Ibid. p. 35.
61. Ibid. p. 105.
62. Ibid.
63. Ibid. p. 37.
64. Ibid. p. 33.
65. Ibid. p. 220.
66. Ibid. p. 31.
67. Ibid. p. 38.
68. Ibid. p. 29.
69. Ibid. p. 376.
70. Haebich, 2000. See note 6.
71. *Bringing Them Home*, 1997, p. 30. See note 1.
72. Cummings, B. (1990). *Take this Child: From Kahlin compound to Retta Dixon Children's Home*. Canberra: Aboriginal Studies Press.
73. Burke, E. (1993). The First Australians: Kinship, family and identity. *Family Matters*, 35 4–6; Heath, F., Bor, W., Thompson, J. & Ox, L. (2011). Diversity, disruption, continuity: Parenting and social and emotional wellbeing amongst Aboriginal peoples and Torres Strait Islanders. *Australian and New Zealand Journal of Family Therapy*, 32 (4) 300–313.
74. Keller, H., Lohaus, A., Kuensemueller, P., Abels, M., Yovsi, R., Voelker, S. & Kulks, D. (2004). The bio-culture of parenting: Evidence from five cultural communities. *Parenting: Science and Practice*, 4 (1) 25–50.
75. Malin, M. (1996). Raising children the Nunga Aboriginal way. *Family Matters*, 43 (Autumn) 43–47; Malin, M. (Ed.). (1997). *Mrs Eyers is No Ogre: A micro study in the exercise of power*. Canberra: Aboriginal Studies Press.
76. Lee, L., Griffiths, C., Glossop, P. & Eapen, V. (2010). The Boomerangs Parenting Program for Aboriginal parents and their young children. *Australasian Psychiatry*, 18 (6) 527–533.
77. Department of Families, Housing, Community Services and Indigenous Affairs (2008). *Occasional Paper 20: Stories on 'growing up' from Indigenous people in the ACT metro/Queanbeyan region*. Canberra: Commonwealth of Australia.
78. Burke, 1993. See note 73.
79. Kruske, S., Belton, S., Wardaguga, M. & Narjic, C. (2012). Growing up our way: The first year of life in remote Aboriginal Australia. *Qualitative Health Research*, 22 (6) 777–787.
80. Goodnow, J. J., Ashmore, J. A., Cotton, S. & Knight, R. (1984). Mothers' developmental timetables in two cultural groups. *International Journal of Psychology*, 19 (3) 193–205.
81. Byers, L., Kulitja, S., Lowell, A. & Kruske, S. (2012). 'Hear our stories': Child-rearing practices of a remote Australian Aboriginal community. *Australian Journal of Rural Health*, 20 (6) 293–297.
82. Ibid.
83. Malin, M. (1996). Raising children the Nunga Aboriginal way. *Family Matters*, 43 (Autumn) 43–47; Nelson, A., Allison, H. & Copley, J. (2007). Understanding where we come from: Occupational therapy with urban Indigenous Australians. *Australian Occupational Therapy Journal*, 54 (3) 203–214.
84. Broome, 1982. See note 22.

85. Kruske et al, 2012, p. 777. See note 79.
86. Atkinson, J., Nelson, J., Brooks, R., Atkinson, C. & Kelleig, R. (2014). Addressing individual trauma and transgenerational trauma. In Dudgeon, P., Milroy, H. & Walker, R. (Eds) (2014). *Working Together: Aboriginal and Torres Strait Islander mental health and wellbeing principles and practice* (2nd edition) (pp. 289–306). Canberra: Commonwealth of Australia, p. 292.
87. Becker, D. (2003). Mental health and human rights: Thinking about the relatedness of individual and social processes. Paper presented at the international conference Towards a Better Future... Building Healthy Communities, 1–3 October 2003, Belfast; Peeters, et al, 2014, p. 171. See note 53.
88. Milroy, H., Dudgeon, P. & Walker, R. (2014). Community life and development programs: Pathways to healing. In *Working Together: Aboriginal and Torres Strait Islander mental health and wellbeing principles and practice* (2nd edition) (pp. 419–435). Canberra: Commonwealth of Australia, p. 419.
89. Dudgeon, P., Walker, R., Scrine, C., Cox, K., D'Anna, D., Dunkley, C., Kelly, K. & Hams, K. (2014). Enhancing wellbeing, empowerment, healing and leadership. In Dudgeon, P., Milroy, H. & Walker, R. (Eds) (2014). *Working Together: Aboriginal and Torres Strait Islander mental health and wellbeing principles and practice* (2nd edition) (pp. 437–448). Canberra: Commonwealth of Australia.
90. Milroy et al, 2014, p. 434. See note 88.
91. Dudgeon et al, 2014, p. 440. See note 89.
92. Peeters quoted in Dudgeon et al, 2014, p. 441. See note 89.
93. Peeters et al, 2014, p. 500. See note 53.
94. Dudgeon et al, 2014, p. 441. See note 89.
95. Peeters et al, 2014, p. 500. See note 53.

Chapter 4
Children and austerity

Carl Harris

I am writing this chapter as a community psychologist – a psychologist with an interest in the fit between the person and their environment. I am informed by my practice as a clinical psychologist working with children and families but also by colleagues in related disciplines. Much of my experience of the impact of the environment on children and families comes from my time working in a number of housing estates in the south of Birmingham.

These estates were originally built as council estates offering low cost rented social housing for working class people. For the last 30 years, in the drive towards a property-owning democracy, UK residents have had the right to buy their council houses. As a consequence, councils have stopped building houses for rent and those in need of social housing have increasingly become those with the least resources. This has changed the nature of these estates and they have become concentrations of multiple layers of deprivation.[1]

Over the same period there has been a significant cultural and social change within the UK. Since the end of the 1970s our working classes have been consistently cast in a critical light. The strength of the structures that protected their rights has been consistently diminished through changes in legislation during Conservative, New Labour and Coalition administrations. The high esteem in which such workers were previously held has been significantly reduced.[2,3] The assault on more communitarian values has been made easier by the presence of beliefs in our culture that justify injustice and inequality: elitism is efficient, exclusion is necessary, prejudice is natural, greed is good and despair is inevitable.[4]

Throughout this period of the introduction of what are described as neoliberal policies, the gap between the richest and poorest sections of our society has grown.[5] This is a pattern that can be seen repeating itself on a global scale. Countries that have introduced such policies (privatisation of national utilities, deregulation and cuts to social spending) have seen the same effect on the distribution of wealth in their society. Such policies have often been introduced during the unstable period that often follows a 'crisis': for example, the Miners' Strike in the UK.[6] Austerity, the period of public spending cuts instigated since the 2010 election, is a new wave of neoliberalism arriving in the wake of the 2008 financial crisis.

Why should we be concerned about this? Well, the social determinants of health – which include social class, poverty, unemployment and poor housing – have been well documented. These determinants ensure that those in the highest social class will, on average, live for eight years longer and enjoy 17 more years without disability than those in the lowest social class.[7] These differences also show themselves very clearly in terms of the different rates of child development between different socioeconomic groups.[8] Neoliberalism means that the social gradient will be steepened and the experiences of the richest and poorest in our society will be increasingly different.

This inequality has damaging effects for society as a whole. The overall levels of social inequality in developed societies – in other words, the size of the gap between the rich and the poor – is correlated with poorer outcomes for the population as a whole. These outcomes include life expectancy and physical health as well as a range of psychologically relevant issues, including mental health problems, drug abuse, interpersonal violence, educational attainment and child wellbeing.[9] This helps us to understand how the UK, the fourth most unequal society in the developed world in terms of income, performs less well than its relative wealth would lead us to expect.[10] The UK is ranked consistently low among developed countries in terms of child wellbeing: twenty-first out of 21 in 2007 and sixteenth out of 29 in 2013.[11,12] Unicef UK has warned that government funding cuts are likely to reverse the relative progress made between these periods.[13]

The environmental influences on human development are vast, varied and complex. This chapter can only begin to describe how austerity interacts with them. In order to do so I will make use of the work of the psychologist Urie Bronfenbrenner.[14] Bronfenbrenner's levels of systems emphasise the role of context. They are a useful way of linking the structures that extend from those people and experiences close to us in our day-to-day lives to the wider social and global systems that influence our development in less obvious ways. His model views each person not as an isolated unit, but as one element in a set of nested social and cultural *systems*, with the largest often having the biggest influence. These are summarised below.

- **Macro level:** on a larger scale determining the prevailing ideology and social structure within which the individual person and his/her micro-, meso- and exo-level systems operate (e.g. current rate of unemployment, other conditions of the labour market, gender roles in society, government policy of austerity).
- **Exo level:** influences on the person and the person's micro- and meso-level systems but of which the person has no direct experience (e.g. a school governing body, a parent's place of work, the local authority's housing department).
- **Meso level:** consisting of two or more of a person's micro-level systems and the links between them (e.g. home–school, hospital–patient's family, mother's family–father's family after separation).
- **Micro level:** of which the individual has regular direct experience (e.g. home, school, work group, club).[15]

At the macro level

At the macro level it is the budget cuts, their impact and the way in which they are justified that are of particular interest. These cuts are large and are impacting upon those who are already experiencing adversity.

In 2012 the Institute for Fiscal Studies (IFS) stated that as a result of coalition policies the numbers in absolute poverty were increasing, and that those in relative poverty would increase after 2013:

> The largest average losses from the 2012–13 reforms as a percentage of income will be among those in the bottom half of the income distribution. Households with children are set to lose the most from the reforms.[16]
>
> In 2012–13 the coalition reforms will increase the numbers of children in absolute/relative poverty by about 200,000/100,000. In 2013–14 the numbers of children in absolute/relative poverty will increase by about 300,000/200,000.[17]

Councils had their government grant cut by 26 per cent over the four years up to 2014, compared with reductions in central government budgets of eight per cent. The funding cuts for charities are similar:

> By the end of the Spending Review period 2015/16, the sector will have lost £1.2 billion in government income each year, a cumulative total of £3.3 billion (NCVO, 2012). Nine out of 10 charities say they are facing 'a riskier future' and spending on children's social care was expected to reduce by an average of 24 per cent in 2011/12.[18]

The number of vulnerable families with children will grow and the measures put in place to mitigate the impact of the recession (such as the Pupil Premium and the Troubled Families Programme) are insufficient to offset its financial effects. These financial effects are exacerbated by the disproportionately high use such families make of services provided by local authorities, which are being reduced through the austerity programme.[19]

These cuts have been facilitated by the austerity narrative that they are a means of correcting the budget deficit which was itself the result of profligate spending by the previous government. This message is highly organised in its development and its repeated, confident delivery by a number of spokespeople in powerful social positions.[20] Austerity's message removes the behaviour of the global banking sector from the narrative and maintains the position that those who have argued for deregulation (and thereby created the conditions that facilitated the crisis) should still be seen as the guardians of our economic future.[21] As part of this narrative, families who claim benefits are presented as undeserving. These families are being subjected to a negative, global judgement by a socially significant authority, while also having few options to improve their circumstances.[22] This approach focuses attention on the behaviour of those who are most disadvantaged, distracting attention from those who are well-off and accumulating an increasing share of society's wealth.

The UK government has acknowledged that it has deficits in its understanding of the perspectives of children in poverty and needs help from others to close this gap in understanding. During the discussion of the Child Poverty Bill, at the committee stage (3 December 2009) Steve Webb (MP for Northavon) wanted to ensure that the government would have to consult children in poverty on any proposals to address child poverty. Helen Goodman (replying for the government) replied,

> While we want to ensure that both the local and national strategies are informed by the views of children and young people, we acknowledge ... that Government may not always be best placed to achieve this goal. In reaching the most disaffected children or those with complex needs, we want to work with those organisations that represent groups that do not usually take part in Government consultations, and that have the necessary specialist skills.[23]

Actions taken since then suggest that the government has little interest in working with such groups or organisations.

New Labour were initially concerned with the issue of 'social exclusion'. As time went by, however, they began to focus their attention on the socially excluded themselves, their characteristics and their use of services. The Coalition continued this process. For instance, they focused on 120,000 'troubled families' and the costs they inflict on society. This figure came from a Social Exclusion Task Force (2007) study, *Families at Risk: Background on families with multiple disadvantages*.[24] While these families were originally represented as experiencing difficulties, they were subsequently presented as causing difficulties. They were both troubled and troubling (to their communities and society). These families are construed as the cause of their own difficulties, along with a welfare state that encourages them to stay at home rather than work. 'Unemployment and benefit dependency are thus defined, even in the context of rapidly rising unemployment, as pathological behaviours on the part of individuals.'[25]

The same process, of shifting focus from structural factors to the moral behaviour of individuals and families, can be seen in apparently even the most benign of government policies – early intervention to prevent damage to the infant's early relationships and developing brain. Early intervention is presented as the solution to the problem of social breakdown:

> The Early Intervention objective is nothing less than to replace a vicious cycle with a virtuous circle; to help every child become a capable and responsible parent who in turn will raise better children who themselves will learn, attain and raise functional families of their own ... We respectfully confront those of all political persuasions with a choice: either we go on trying to patch up the consequences of social breakdown or we tackle the roots and the transmission of underachievement.[26]

This moral narrative is supported by the partial view of neurodevelopmental research presented in the report sponsored by Graham Allen MP.[27,28] The moral and neurological development of the child, in a time of austerity, becomes a vehicle for blaming the poor. There is a consensus across the mainstream political spectrum around the impact of parenting on the development of the child. There is little recognition, however, of the factors that mean that some families are more focused on getting by than others. This message is also at odds with the evidence: most people in poverty now come from working households due to low wages and the increasing cost of living.[29]

Children in austerity are presented as the victims of their parents' behaviour towards them. By decontextualising such children and their parents from the structural context of poverty and unemployment, austerity rhetoric renders them appropriate for modular interventions which focus on their behaviours rather than considering the wider determinants of their circumstances.

At the exo level

The exo level refers to elements of our ecosystem that influence our lives but with which we do not have contact. Public access to one of these spaces opened briefly on a Saturday morning on 24 October 2014 – a demonstration in Birmingham city centre in support of the Youth Service. Youth workers attended the demonstration accompanying members of their client groups. Many young people performed and had the opportunity to voice their opinion on the threatened cuts to their services. The practitioners attending stepped outside the 'normal' environment and their expected role in relation to the young people. They had the opportunity to engage in a shared, supportive space with others from similar occupational niches but also with others, such as politicians, activists and members of the public.

A number of Labour councillors spoke of the need to make the Youth Service a statutory service. One of the politicians' speeches was made by a Labour MP. He spoke of how a local Conservative councillor had told a local police inspector that there were a lot of problems with the youth in his constituency. He described how the inspector had said that he disagreed with this, saying that young people were a community with which the police needed to engage. He then described decisions taken in Westminster by politicians who did not understand the importance of the Youth Service to young people who had suffered disadvantage. Using expletives he went on to describe those ministers who had made these decisions. An activist who was moving through the crowd selling the *Socialist Worker* commented, 'That's all very well but they [Labour] are still signed up to austerity.'

The message from the young people who took to the stage to explain the importance of the Youth Service in their lives was very clear:

> We need somewhere safe to go and hang out with our friends, especially in the winter. If we don't have somewhere to go we end up hanging around on the streets and trouble finds us ... The youth workers who support us don't just play pool with us. They listen to us, they support us to find jobs or get qualifications. They help to build our confidence. They are like family.

Two young boys from the estates in the south of the city both rapped. Their words are presented later in the chapter. Their raps are an outcome of their interaction with their local Youth Service. Their words help us understand how the support of the service helped them to express themselves. They are also a direct comment on the social circumstances in which they find themselves.

As part of the research for this chapter, I met with the two directors of an innovative, local project training social work students. This project was set up in March 2010 following the council's decision to equalise the distribution of family support across the city. This had meant, in the south of the city, that one provider had to provide support for families across a much wider area than before. This change had meant the loss of capacity in terms of (amongst other things) staff, goodwill, local knowledge and relationships. The two originators of the project had used student social work placement funding from local universities to provide a social work/family support service to those families living in the council estates in the south of the city. The project had responded in a creative, thoughtful way to the demands of austerity and the needs of the families in their area – an innovative response to austerity. This had required a significant risk on the part of the two originators and an ongoing commitment on their part, which sometimes meant that they didn't take a salary.

The project had been given a Big Society Award in the early days of the Coalition government. It had managed to survive the first impact of austerity but had been affected by the cuts to their purchasers' budgets (i.e. universities and colleges providing social work qualifications). This funding was reduced recently, with just 12 weeks' notice, meaning an £800 shortfall in funding per student and a £100,000 funding gap per annum for the project as a whole. This reduction would not appear as a direct cut in a service. It would be seen as a cut in education funding. The money had been working very hard both for students and for the families who benefited from their support. Austerity had meant that the funding for one activity had become 'built in' to the funding for another. A cut in funding for an educational enterprise had become a cut in service to a population who had already lost their initial service.

As a consequence of both increased family difficulties and reduced non-statutory supports, the demand for the service was escalating. Caseloads for the students on placement had more than doubled and there was now a waiting list for the service. This is a picture that is repeated across the vast majority of such services in the country. The project management team have had to start diverting some of their capacity to the identification of other funding sources. As qualified social workers themselves they provide supervision and support to the trainees but they are less available to do this while they are carrying out scoping activities. Cuts to Legal Aid have meant that they have been unable to formalise living arrangements for a young girl they have been working with and who now lives with her grandmother. As predicted by the Office of the Children's Commissioner, these changes to Legal Aid have meant a 'negative effect on affected children and young people by curtailing their access to justice … and skilled and appropriate representation'. The government did little to assess the impact of the changes on children and young people.[30] The lack of availability of legal support has certainly had an impact on this family's access to financial support.

Another important part of the exo level is the co-ordination local authorities provide within their locality. This is crucial to plans to roll out free nursery places. There are significant barriers to the success of this policy. Families in disadvantaged areas often do not access childcare because they are not aware of it, don't access information about it, or have an inaccurate understanding of its cost. For the effective roll-out of free provision for two-year-olds, local authorities will have to support providers in overcoming barriers to access for the families most in need.[31]

There are also barriers from the providers' side. Childcare providers in disadvantaged areas are highly reliant on funded places as there is low demand for paid-for places. Achieving sustainability in disadvantaged areas is made harder still by the transient nature of the population. For childcare to be sustainable in disadvantaged areas it will need to be publicly funded in one form or another. Private providers will also need councils to provide free staff training to ensure that the child care provided is of high quality.[32] While childcare in the UK is provided through a free market, this market will fail to deliver to those most in need without local authority support.

At the meso level

The meso system is where micro-systems interact. This typically refers to a neighbourhood, where children and families mingle both in and out of school, work, local shops and households. Austerity increases the wealth disparities in our society and degrades the public institutions which provide our shared social environments. As a consequence, deprived neighbourhoods and those who live in them are becoming increasingly neglected and marginalised.[33] For children such neighbourhoods can be intimidating and inhospitable environments, not places where they feel free to play in safety. For young people, feeling safe often involves gathering in groups in public spaces. This behaviour is then experienced as intimidating by others, creating more tension between those who inhabit this shared space.[34]

Those living in the estates are often sceptical of the notion that they are socially excluded. They can, however, identify the judgements that others make of them. These judgements become an 'invisible barrier' to their participation outside their normal space. In Lisa McKenzie's *Getting By* a female lone parent from an estate in Nottingham describes how the prejudice shows itself in the pause an official makes when recording her details: 'I know what they're thinking; you can see it ticking over in their brain as you wait for them to think "oh it's one of them from there."'[35] Feeling 'out of place' and 'looked down on' makes it difficult to leave the estate. The estate then becomes a place of identity, a place of safety at the same time as being a source of stigma. The estate offers safety from the experience of being looked down on. The estate itself is not physically safe, although you are safer if you are integrated, if you fit in, if you are known and connected within it.

For McKenzie this creates 'estatism':[36] 'Through fear of not knowing how you may be treated and viewed by unknown others, unhealthy emotional attachments are made to a neighbourhood, particularly by the young, making it more difficult to make positive networks outside of the estate but also within it.'[37] The austerity narrative focuses attention on the behaviour of those who find it difficult to leave the estate rather than on those making such judgements. The narrative also gives permission to people to make those judgements and increases the barriers still further.

As part of its response to austerity, the local authority in Birmingham has begun a process of 'asset transfer'. Facilities that it no longer has the capacity to maintain are being offered to other organisations on the understanding that they will maintain them and use them for local people. One such building is a local community hall. Two local community project volunteers attended a meeting with members of the local authority to determine whether they would be allowed to take on the running of the hall. The volunteers referred to this as a 'liability transfer'. The hall, being more than 40 years old, is a building with problems. These problems include a heating system that produces heating bills that could bankrupt the community project and which the project does not have the resources to replace. The project team want to keep rates low for users of the hall so that leisure activities are available locally – an important support to local children's experience of social inclusion. The local children's centre also uses the hall to provide outreach support to those who would not travel across the estate to make use of its facilities. The stay and play sessions often have to be cancelled in winter, however, as the hall is too cold. Each such cancellation means a reduction in service but also a reduction in the confidence of local families that it is worth getting out of the house to go to the hall. This means fewer interactions between families and children, and fewer opportunities for mutual support.

A local, newly formed church is a regular user of the hall. Its members come from outside the estates and are of relatively high socioeconomic status. To advertise their weekly worship they placed a large banner on the fence around the hall. The community workers reported that residents appeared to see this as a sign that the hall had become a church and assumed that it was no longer available to them. The workers have asked that the banner only be put up on days of services.

Austerity has had an impact on local people's access to the hall and to interactions between family groups. Heating the hall presents a financial threat to the project, whose workers now spend more of their time looking for solutions to the financial threat and less time promoting use of the hall. The financial consequences may include increasing rates for hire, which would increase the financial barrier for local groups and reduce participation in affordable activities. The capacity of the meso level to support interactions between families (micro-level systems) has been reduced. The 'contested ownership' of the hall disturbed people's perceptions of the availability of the hall for public use. Residents revised their 'mental maps' of their area and removed one of the safe spaces where they could take their children. While this misconception was swiftly corrected it demonstrated a belief that local resources were not permanently available and could be removed with no consultation or notice. This tells us about residents' experience of the availability of local resources in the past as well as how this experience informs their expectations of the future. This is the framework into which austerity presents itself and within which children develop their expectations of their neighbourhood in the future.

In the local estate in 2011–12, 17 per cent of the local secondary school pupils achieved five or more A* to C grade passes at GCSE, compared with a national average of 59 per cent. Environmental factors account for the majority of this difference. Estates where deprivation is concentrated in layers that interact and compound each other's effects are stressful places to live. Children who live amongst transient neighbours and classmates, sleep in bedrooms affected by damp, and are surrounded by signs of social disorder like graffiti and broken windows show chronically raised levels of the stress hormone cortisol. This places them at risk of ill health but also compromises their ability to learn and remember.[38] Austerity compounds these difficulties but also affects the degree to which school is a support to children and exacerbates the influence of social class on children's experience.[39] In congruence with neoliberal market ideology, middle-class parents perceive themselves as consumers of services. They can help their child's teacher to understand their child's needs and their vision of their child's future using language and terminology with which the teacher will be familiar. They and the teacher can then bring this future into the present when they discuss the meaning of the child's actions.[40] Working-class parents, on the other hand, are more likely to describe themselves as clients of services, becoming involved when there are difficulties with their child's behaviour or academic performance.[41] Early childhood educators and childcare providers are well aware of the impact of socioeconomic issues on academic outcomes and yet they do not often consider poverty as an issue when they consider the outcomes of the children they work with. In line with the narrative of austerity, these practitioners tend to see poverty as the fault of those who experience it. This tends to make practitioners less co-constructive – a very different relationship to that which middle-class parents experience.[42]

Estates have become places where disadvantage and deprivation are increasingly concentrated – a process that has been exacerbated by austerity. This means that those who live there are already exposed to a set of community and neighbourhood risk factors which will impact upon them as families and individuals. The resources available to them to manage these risks are becoming fewer, less available, less supportive and harder-pressed as a result of austerity.

At the micro level

At the micro level children spend most of their time within the family system. Families are living increasingly precarious lives, with jobs, income and accommodation all less secure. Parents are under constant strain as they live with the threat of unexpected financial shocks. Austerity is increasing the number of children living in poverty, which exposes families to a greater number of stressors. Poverty also increases the negative effects of the stressors that families experience.[43] Poverty creates a 'context of stress', which can include conflict, food insecurity and residential mobility.[44] Such a stressful family environment is a clear marker of potential mental health difficulties for children.[45] When parents are stressed, children are likely to be stressed.

Families are being expected to absorb the risks from which they had been previously buffered by elements of our fiscal and welfare systems. As austerity attacks the public sector, the protective elements of our institutions are being dismantled, and those in poverty, those who do not own property, and those who do not have a permanent contract with fixed terms and hours are being expected to manage the risks inherent in having a more 'flexible' economy and workforce. Low wages and long hours mean that parents in British families appear to be more time-pressured than other countries in Europe.[46] Because wages are low, families' incomes are also determined by the calculations made by the tax credit and benefits system. This means constantly monitoring spending but with less ability to predict income in the next week, let alone the next months or years. Families are only one unexpected bill away from financial crisis. Without savings, they rely on borrowing from family and friends.[47]

Children are very aware of their family's financial circumstances and of the effect of these problems on their parents. They will also notice the difference if their parent manages to find work. They notice that the family has more money and more access to goods and activities than previously. They will also, however, be aware of the impact of work on their parent's wellbeing, especially if they are in a single-parent household. Children will still be anxious about money, especially if the employment is temporary, as is frequently the case.[48] Children are affected directly by poverty, in some cases going without food, bedding or heating, but also indirectly through its impact on their family and parents. Children find ways to address the impact of poverty on themselves and their families but even these solutions introduce new tensions as they try to reconcile the demands that different micro-level systems place upon them (e.g. home, work and school).[49] Children have to reconcile themselves to not being able to have particular things. They may conceal such needs in order to reduce family or parental stress. They may not mention a school trip, judging that it will be unaffordable and thereby excluding themselves from the activity. They may find a job to help them participate in their social networks and make and sustain friendships. This can, however, create tensions with satisfying the requirements of school.[50]

Materialism is of particular significance for British families' experience of inequality. While Swedish families are more likely to see inequality in terms of access to outdoor activities and Spanish families more in terms of contact with the extended family, British families are more likely to think of inequality in terms of material possessions. British parents are also more likely to promote the acquisition of new toys and technological gadgets than other parents in Europe.[51] Children in different social classes in different European countries tend to downplay the importance of material possessions for their wellbeing. The exception seems to be British children living in poverty. For them, possessions seem to play an important role in social inclusion. They may well be using possession of these items as a means of covering up feelings of shame and inadequacy. Materialism and austerity are a toxic combination for these children: not having the key symbolic markers of social inclusion – the right phone or the right trainers – means marginalisation and even bullying.[52]

Poverty impacts on children's participation in another important micro-level system – school – in a number of ways. They can't afford the materials that are expected at school, they often can't afford to go on school trips and they can't always afford the correct uniform, so find themselves involved in disciplinary action. These children also notice that they are treated differently by teachers and pupils alike. They often feel discriminated against by teachers and, lacking the symbolic possessions of social inclusion, can be bullied by other children.[53] These factors can have a significant effect on school attendance. Such social exclusion means anxiety, unhappiness and social insecurity. The narrative of austerity means that, even if these children were to acquire such items, their actions would be seen as evidence that they are not truly poor. These judgements, facilitated by the austerity narrative and made with little understanding of the meaning of the item for the child, further exclude children in poverty.

As the risk factors impacting on families increase and the supports available to them reduce, so the burden children have to bear will increase. Under austerity children are more likely to have to bear some of the family's financial burden. In such circumstances the resources of the family become redistributed. The children will often take on more responsibilities and may take on the care of siblings. They may have to take on the care of an adult with physical or mental health difficulties. Children in this young carer role are often cut off from shared activities with other children, especially as the organisations providing this support have reduced capacity.

More families now live in private rented – rather than local authority – accommodation. Their living circumstances have become more precarious and austerity has made this worse. Families are more likely to have to move, with a knock-on effect for their children's connections with friends and school. Such moves mean that energy will have to be invested in rebuilding these networks in the new environment, reducing the energy left for engaging with academic attainment.

Experiencing stress in childhood is problematic in itself but can also lead to sensitivity to stress over the whole life course. Adults who experienced psychological stress as children show increased levels of cortisol in their bloodstream throughout their life.[54] Children born into poverty will consequently experience more illness and live a shorter life. They will also be at increased risk of other threats to life and health. Being in a household with greater levels of stress means a child will find it more difficult to concentrate and succeed academically. This will make it less likely that they will attain higher socioeconomic status and enjoy the corresponding wellbeing. Their emotional development may also be adversely affected, making them less likely to be able to form satisfying relationships and enjoy the health-sustaining benefits of social support.[55]

The raps

James's words

> My dad's in prison not just for one reason
> made many mistakes all for no reason
> hope he stays in 48 seasons
> thro' away the key and leave him
> it ent slapstick it takes practice

> to spit these bars and perfect these tactics
> drop these bars rap them up package
> send it off MCs try to hack it
> find your own bars go practice
> i'll do my own thing hat-trick
> I'm a lyrical miracle I'm on fire
> bars I'm spitting making me higher
> it's fire when I'm in the bouf
> no fiction the truth try spit these bars
> you may lose a tooth

James begins his piece by describing his circumstances and his family's experience. He goes on to say that expressing yourself in this way is not easy: 'it ent slapstick it takes practice, to spit these bars and perfect these tactics.' He has had to work hard to learn how to use words in this format: 'drop these bars rap them up package, send it off' and then to perform the material in front of an audience. This requires discipline and commitment and an ability to talk about personal experiences in front of people who are not known to him.

When we met to discuss using his rap in this chapter, James spoke about how the rap 'comes from inside': it is his material and he feels a personal connection to it. He made it clear that this work is owned by him and he gives this message in the rap itself: 'send it off MCs [microphone controllers] try to hack it, find your own bars go practice.' In their raps both James and Jake refer to MCs as people who are the mouthpieces for their group or community.

The last section of the rap describes how powerful James has found the experience of writing and performing in this way. In his description he uses the phrase 'lyrical miracle' and talks about how the act of performing makes him feel: 'bars I'm spitting making me higher.' The experience of delivering his account of how-things-really-are is an empowering and liberating one for him. This is an endorsement of the Youth Service that has supported him in expressing himself in this way. He finishes with a warning: 'no fiction the truth try spit these bars, you may lose a tooth.' As before James talks about how he has to 'spit these bars': they have to be delivered with a personal commitment and passion. There is a risk to this though: 'you may lose a tooth.' This could be a warning to anybody who wants to steal his material, or it could be a statement about how talking in this way and speaking the truth carries an element of risk.

Jake's words

> Fuck staying at the bottom I'm a win this election
> politicians feed the people's minds with deception
> cos they don't have a chance to share their perception
> in the USA cops shot a youth cos he shot a weapon
> is it lies or an official gang?
> conspiracy fearers are lies as government slang
> he had his hands on his phone and a wallet in his hand
> these MCs bite out corruption like a fang
> they say they'll make a change to make votes
> all their policies sink like titanic boats
> will they ever make a government make a parliament that will float
> they don't care for people
> they just want money n that's the root of all evil
> things become old medieval
> so I keep my bars straight up nothing deceitful

Jake's rap begins with a statement about how he sees his position, and uses a political metaphor for how he intends to change the situation. He then goes on to describe how he sees the current political system. He sees politicians lying to the people and the people having no opportunity to share their view of what is happening. Jake uses an example of this: there have been some highly publicised shootings of black youths in the USA. He describes how difficult it is to trust the official account of any such incident. He asks us to consider whether any report of such an incident is simply 'lies or an official gang conspiracy'. Jake talks about 'conspiracy fearers'; these may be people who are uncertain whom to believe and who wonder whether some group or other in society is acting on their own agenda in a secret plan co-ordinated with many others. If so, this could refer to the police or the government, or to an 'unofficial' group, such as a gang.

By describing government communication as 'slang' in this way Jake makes the point that all information is produced and authorised by one social group or another to present their own version of events. The government's communications can be as difficult for outsiders to understand as any other 'insider' terminology. Referring to this communication as slang, Jake 'equalises' the authority of government and non-government accounts.

He then returns to the details of the shooting where the information about the youth's behaviour is at odds with the official version of events.

The police said that he shot a weapon but other accounts described how 'he had his hands on his phone and a wallet in his hand'. Jake refers to the MCs who will challenge any corruption in the official version of events. The MCs are a source of truth. Jake brings political activity back into focus. He describes politicians as saying 'they'll make a change' but this is only to secure votes. In his description their words are a tool for gaining support but 'all their policies sink like titanic boats'. The sinking of the Titanic showed how disasters impact on different classes to a greater or lesser extent. In the first-class sections of the ship, 97 per cent of women and children survived, compared with 42 per cent of women and children in third class. The inquiry by Lord Mersey concluded that there had been no policy of preventing third-class passengers from accessing the lifeboats but there were no passengers from third class called as witnesses to the inquiry.[56] Nevertheless, Lord Mersey concluded:

> It is no doubt true that the proportion of third-class passengers saved falls far short of the proportion of the first and second class, but this is accounted for by the greater reluctance of the third-class passengers to leave the ship, by their unwillingness to part with their baggage, by the difficulty in getting them up from their quarters, which were at the extreme ends of the ship, and by other similar causes.[57]

The design of the ship was notoriously complicated, making it very difficult to get out of the third-class accommodation. This resonates with the low and declining levels of social mobility in the UK.[58] Lord Mersey makes reference to this but also to the behaviour of those in third class. Are those in third class being blamed for their own loss of life? If the account of their behaviour is accurate, is it understandable that they would be reluctant to leave their possessions?

Jake argues that politicians are motivated by their own material self-interest. His words relate to a verse in Timothy Chapter 6, Verse 10: 'For the love of money is the root of all evil'[59] – a phrase with powerful social resonances. Jake's reference to 'things become old medieval' notes that human experience in this country was harsher in previous times before the rule of law. Yet, for some, the rule of law is less applicable in their day-to-day existence.

At the end Jake notes, as did James, that the words he says are the truth. He distinguishes himself from those who tell lies. He and James are MCs; according to the rules of their community, their words can be trusted and are not influenced by those in authority. Jake is describing how he is distanced from those who hold political power. He does not feel they can be trusted and believes that they will distort the truth for their own narrow self-interest. Austerity is increasing the distance between James and Jake and the politicians they criticise, but for Jake and James it is this distance that gives their words authenticity. James and Jake have expressed themselves in their raps, given words to the powerful feelings they experience as a result of their circumstances. They have then taken their work and performed it in a city centre venue in front of a crowd which included an MP. Their efforts, combined with those of the youth workers who supported them in this process, have closed the gap between them and those who are in a position to influence their life experience.

The gap, however, remains huge, and is growing.

Endnotes

1. Minton, A. (2012). *Ground Control: Fear and happiness in the twenty-first-century city*. London: Penguin.
2. Jones, O. (2012). *Chavs: The demonization of the working class*. London: Verso Books.
3. McKenzie, L. (2015). *Getting By: Estates, class and culture in austerity Britain*. Bristol: Policy Press.
4. Dorling, D. (2011). *Injustice: Why social inequality persists*: Bristol: Policy Press.
5. Harvey, D. (2005). *A Brief History of Neoliberalism*. Oxford: Oxford University Press.
6. Klein, N. (2008). *The Shock Doctrine: The rise of disaster capitalism*. London: Penguin.
7. Marmot, M. (2010). *Fair Society, Healthy Lives: The Marmot Review*. London: The Marmot Review.
8. Feinstein, L. (2003). Inequality in the early cognitive development of British children in the 1970 cohort. *Economica, 70* (277) 73–97.
9. Wilkinson, R. & Pickett, K. (2009). *The Spirit Level: Why more equal societies almost always do better*. London: Allen Lane.
10. Dorling, D. (2011). *Injustice: Why social inequality persists*: Bristol: Policy Press.
11. UNICEF (2007). *Child Poverty in Perspective: An overview of child well-being in rich countries* (Innocenti Report Card 7). Florence: UNICEF Innocenti Research Centre.
12. UNICEF (2013). *Child Well-being in Rich Countries: A comparative overview* (Innocenti Report Card 11). Florence: UNICEF Office of Research.
13. BBC News (2013). UK rises up Unicef child well-being ranking. Available at http://www.bbc.co.uk/news/uk-22083762 (retrieved June 2015).
14. Bronfenbrenner, U. (1979). *The Ecology of Human Development: Experiments by nature and design*. Cambridge, MA: Harvard University Press.
15. Orford, J. (1992). *Community Psychology: Theory and practice*. Chichester: Wiley.
16. Joyce, R. (2012). *Tax and Benefit Reforms Due in 2012–13, and the Outlook for Household Incomes* (IFS Briefing Note 126). London: Institute for Fiscal Studies, p. 17.
17. Brewer, M. & Joyce, R. (2013). *Child and Working-age Poverty to 2013–14* (IFS Briefing

Note 115). London: Institute of Financial Studies, p. 3.
18. Action for Children (2012). *The Red Book: As long as it takes*. London: Action for Children, p. 11.
19. Reed, H. (2012). *In the Eye of the Storm: Britain's forgotten children and families. A research report for Action for Children*. London: The Children's Society and NSPCC.
20. Afoko, C. & Vockins, D. (2013). *Framing the Economy: The austerity story*. London: New Economics Foundation.
21. Touraine, A. (2014). *After the Crisis*. Cambridge: Polity Press.
22. Harkness, S., Gregg, P. & MacMillan, L. (2012). *Poverty: The role of institutions, behaviours and culture*. York: Joseph Rowntree Foundation.
23. House of Commons (2009). *Child Poverty Bill: Committee stage report*. Bill No. 10 of 2009-10. Research Paper 09/89, p. 15.
24. Social Exclusion Task Force (2007). *Families at Risk: Background on families with multiple disadvantages*. London: Cabinet Office.
25. Levitas, R. (2012) *There May Be 'Trouble' Ahead: What we know about those 120,000 'troubled' families* (Policy Response Series No. 3). Bristol: PSE UK, p. 5.
26. Allen, G. & Duncan Smith, I. (2008). *Early Intervention: Good parents, great kids, better citizens*. London: The Centre for Social Justice & The Smith Institute, pp. 6-7.
27. Wastell, D. & White, S. (2012). Blinded by neuroscience: Social policy, the family and the infant brain. *Families, Relationships and Societies*, 1 (3) 397-414.
28. Allen, G. (2011). *Early Intervention the Next Steps*. London: Department for Work and Pensions and Cabinet Office.
29. MacInnes, T., Aldridge, H., Bushe, S., Kenway P. & Tinson, A. (2013). *Monitoring Poverty and Social Exclusion 2013*. York: New Policy Institute for the Joseph Rowntree Foundation.
30. Children's Commissioner (2013). *Office of the Children's Commissioner's response to the Ministry of Justice consultation: Transforming legal aid: Delivering a more credible and efficient system*. London: The Office of the Children's Commissioner.
31. Dickens, S., Wollney, I., & Ireland, E. (2012). *Childcare Sufficiency and Sustainability in Disadvantaged Areas*. London: Department for Education.
32. Ibid.
33. Harris, C. (2014). The impact of austerity on a British council estate. *The Psychologist*, 27 (4) 250-253.
34. Ridge, T. (2011). The everyday costs of poverty in childhood: A review of qualitative research exploring the lives and experiences of low-income children in the UK. *Children and Society*, 25, 73-84.
35. McKenzie, L. (2015). *Getting By: Estates, class and culture in austerity Britain*. Bristol: Policy Press, p. 73.
36. Hanley, L. (2007). *Estates: An intimate history*. London: Granta.
37. McKenzie, 2015, p. 162. See note 35.
38. Wilkinson, R. & Pickett, K. (2009). *The Spirit Level: Why more equal societies almost always do better*. London: Allen Lane.
39. Gillies, V. & Edwards, R. (2011). Clients or consumers, commonplace or pioneers? Navigating the contemporary class politics of family, parenting skills and education. *Ethics and Education* 6 (2) 141.
40. Panofsky, C. P. & Vadeboncoeur, J. A. (2012). Schooling the social classes: Triadic zones of proximal development, communicative capital, and relational distance in the perpetuation of advantage. In H. Daniels (Ed.). *Vygotsky and Sociology* (pp. 192-210). New York: Routledge.

41. See note 39.
42. Simpson, D., Lumsden, E. & McDowall Clark, R. (2014). Neoliberalism, global poverty policy and early childhood education and care: A critique of local uptake in England. *Early Years: An international research journal, 35* (1) 96–109.
43. DuBois, D. L., Felner, R. D., Meares, H. & Krier, M. (1994). Prospective investigation of the effects of socioeconomic disadvantage, life stress and social support on early adolescent adjustment. *Journal of Abnormal Psychology, 103*, 511–522.
44. McLoyd, V. (1990). The impact of economic hardship on black families and children: Psychological distress, parenting and socioemotional development. *Child Development, 61*, 311–346.
45. Wille, N., Bettge, S. & Ravens-Sieberer, U. (2008). Risk and protective factors for children's and adolescents' mental health: Results of the BELLA study. *European Child and Adolescent Psychiatry, 17*, Supplement 1.
46. Nairn, A. & Ipsos MORI (2011). *Children's Well-being in UK, Sweden and Spain: The role of inequality and materialism.* London: UNICEF and Ipsos MORI Social Research Institute.
47. Action for Children (2013). *The Red Book: Children under pressure.* London: Action for Children.
48. Ridge, T. (2011). The everyday costs of poverty in childhood: A review of qualitative research exploring the lives and experiences of low-income children in the UK. *Children and Society, 25*, 73–84.
49. Ibid.
50. Ibid.
51. See note 46.
52. Ibid.
53. See note 48.
54. Wadsworth, M. E. & Berger, L. E. (2006). Adolescents coping with poverty-related family stress: Prospective predictors of coping and psychological symptoms. *Journal of Youth and Adolescence, 3*, 57–70.
55. Bartley, M. (2012). Life getting under the skin: Childhood stress and adult health. In M. Bartley (Ed.). *Life Gets Under Your Skin* (pp. 16–18). London: UCL Research Department in Epidemiology and Public Health on behalf of ESRC International Centre for Lifecourse Studies in Society and Health.
56. Hall, W. (1986). Social class and survival on the SS Titanic. *Social Science and Medicine, 22* (6) 687–690.
57. Lord Mersey (1912). *British Parliamentary Papers: Shipping casualties (Loss of the Steamship 'Titanic')* cmd. 6352. London: HMSO, p. 40.
58. Dorling, D. (2011). *Injustice: Why social inequality persists*: Bristol: Policy Press.
59. King James Bible, Timothy, 6:10.

Chapter 5
Single motherhood

Laura Golding

The immediate associations that go with the words 'single mother' are often negative. Newspaper headlines frequently shout about the negative impact of single parenthood: 'Children in single parent families "worse behaved",' 'The single mother of eight children planning a lavish Christmas – all funded by benefits worth £2,200 a MONTH,' 'Children in single-parent families more likely to suffer emotional problems, report finds,' and so on.[1,2,3] Indeed, even rather more considered accounts of single motherhood depict a less than positive picture:

> We ... can't take a sick day, and can't take a rest unless our child falls asleep. There is no one to share the enchanting moments and tantrums with, no one to read a book to our child while we have a bath, no one to reassure us that we're doing just fine.[4]

This chapter provides an account of single motherhood and some of its features. It does this from a number of different perspectives. It focuses on the experiences of single mothers as well as the impact of lone parenting on children, covering areas including stigma and shame, poverty, the impact of lone parenting on children's lives, and single motherhood due to bereavement of a partner. It also considers the role of attachment and resilience. This is an account based partly on professional knowledge and the relevant research literature. It also includes a personal perspective and the experiences and views of a range of other single mothers. Some of these are known to me in my personal life or professional life, and others are celebrities whose single mother status is the subject of media attention. The language of this chapter is of mothers and fathers. It is, however, fully acknowledged that separation, divorce and loss of a partner occur in same-sex parental relationships.

It could be argued that everything that is said about single motherhood applies equally to single fatherhood. The more generic term 'lone parent' is commonly used in the media and research literature. However, the majority of lone parents are single mothers. The Office of National Statistics reported that in 2012 only nine per cent of single parents were fathers.[5] Much of the attention of the psychology and psychiatry research literature has been on single mothers. Of course, the reasons for this focus require some examination. Although some of what is described and discussed in this chapter applies to lone parenthood, rather than single motherhood *per se*, the main focus is on the experience of mothers.

Most commonly, women become single mothers due to separation and/or divorce.[6] For others, their single mother status has come about due to the death of their partner. A smaller minority, however, are single mothers by choice – a distinct group who differ in many significant ways from those who become single mothers owing to separation, divorce or death of a partner.[7] This chapter focuses on those for whom their status as single mothers is *not* a choice. The circumstances under which women come to be single mothers not by choice vary. However, there are many ways in which single mothers are connected no matter how they have come to be in this position. In doing some background reading for this chapter, it is striking that, whatever the perspective of what I have read, every article, report or book chapter on single motherhood notes a substantial increase in the number of lone-parent households over the past 40 to 50 years or so, the vast majority of which are headed by single mothers.[8] In the UK lone parents with dependent children represent 26 per cent of all families with dependent children. This has increased by four per cent since 1996.[9] These statistics in themselves challenge the social construct of two parents, one male and one female, being the 'norm'. With lone parents heading one in four households, the norms, as such, appear to be shifting.

In 2012 UK women accounted for 91 per cent of lone parents. This trend is seen in other countries too. For example, in 2006 about 18.3 per cent of all Canadian families were lone-parent households.[10] In 1971 this figure was 9.4 per cent – this, therefore, has nearly doubled in 35 years. In Canada 80 per cent of lone-parent households are headed by mothers.[11] Similar increases in the number of lone-parent households have been seen in the USA and in France.[12,13]

So, what is it like to be a single mother and what impact does single motherhood have on children's lives?

Some facts

Gingerbread, the UK charity that provides advice and support for single parents, provides some sobering statistics.

- There are two million single parents in Britain.
- Fewer than two per cent of single parents are teenagers.
- The median age of single parents is 38.1.
- 23 per cent of all dependent children live in a single parent household.
- Children in single-parent families are twice as likely as children in couple families to live in relative poverty.
- Only two-fifths of single parents receive child support from their child's other parent.[14]

Stigma and shame

Societal stigma relating to single motherhood exists. As one researcher has pointed out, 'the socially constructed ideal of what constitutes good motherhood does not typically evoke images of single mothers.'[15] I have been a single mother (not by choice) since 2009. However, six years on, I rarely describe myself to others as a single mother. Within my professional life I talk about having children but I seldom explicitly come out to colleagues (interestingly, I was going to type here the word 'admit' here) as being a single parent. This is due, in part, to my wish and need to maintain professional boundaries and to keep my private life to myself at work. However, a more honest examination of my decision not to talk about my single mother status tells me that this comes in part from a sense of shame, from a worry that I will be viewed as something other, seen as incomplete and judged negatively. It was instructive, for example, that my immediate feeling, on being invited to write this chapter for this book, was worry: worry that to include my personal perspective on single motherhood would inevitably 'out' me.

Reflecting with other women in the same position on the extent to which we come out to others about our single mother status suggests that I am not alone in feeling like this. Jane, a friend who is a single mother of a teenage daughter, describes avoiding telling others that she is a single mother: 'I also don't "admit", but skirt around the details of my situation instead, hoping people don't ask.' Reflecting on why this may be, Jane wonders if part of the reason for this is a worry about the negative assumptions that others might make:

> I wouldn't say I choose to parent this way but the reasons why I am indicates something's wrong with it ... part of me frets that other people think such things as 'can't hold down a relationship', 'is a flawed person' ... It's easier for people to describe themselves as married and for the listener to not need to ask further questions and just to accept the fact in a positive way, but it's not okay to say 'I'm a single parent' and for the listener to not want to know more details. People usually do, or I need to qualify why I am.

Single mothers' worries about societal stigma with regards to single motherhood are not misplaced. In a survey of 1,500 single parents carried out by Gingerbread in March 2014, 50 per cent of those polled stated that they felt that stigma relating to single parents in the media had increased over the past two years, and 20 per cent believed that there was a greater stigma regarding single parenthood in workplaces and in the wider community. In addition, 75 per cent of parents polled reported personal experience of stigma due to their single-parent status. Examples of this included being refused jobs and regularly reading and hearing negative comments about single parents in the media.[16]

The author J.K. Rowling is one of the most famous single mothers in the UK today. She has spoken eloquently on her experience in the early days of becoming a single mother. She describes how she was perceived by others and how her single parent status appeared to come to define her in a largely negative way:

> My overriding memory of that time is the slowly evaporating sense of self-esteem ... it was slowly dawning on me that I was now defined, in the eyes of many, by something I had never chosen. I was a Single Parent, and a Single Parent On Benefits to boot.[17]

Rowling goes on to describe how her status as a single parent remained a dominant feature when she became famous, as if it still defined her:

> There was still no escaping the Single Parent tag; it followed me to financial stability and fame just as it had clung to me in poverty and obscurity. I became Single Parent Writes Award-Winning Children's Book/Earns Record American Advance/Gets Film Deal.[18]

So it seems that, no matter how we might choose to define ourselves, knowledge that we are single mothers sometimes leads to negative responses and assumptions. Key to this, particularly reflected in the tabloid press, is the supposed link between single mothers and welfare benefit use. Likewise is the misplaced belief that many single mothers are teenagers – in fact, only two per cent of single mothers are teenagers.[19]

My colleague Dorothy has been a single mother of two daughters, now aged 17 and 18, for six years. She recalls making a decision to wear a ring on her wedding finger when going for an interview for a consultant clinical psychologist post. She did this as she was mindful of the stigma of being a single mother:

> I wore a ring on my wedding finger so the assumption would be made that I was married. I knew they couldn't ask me those questions outright but also believed that my marital/parenting status would have a bearing on whether I could undertake a challenging role. I didn't want them to have any doubts about my ability to do the job I was going for.

An article published in *The Guardian* in October 2014 celebrated the bronze sculpture entitled *Real Birmingham Family* created by the Turner Prize-winning artist Gillian Wearing. This depicts two single mothers, one of whom is clearly pregnant. The sculpture shows them walking purposefully whilst holding hands with their two young sons. Lola Okolosie, the author of the newspaper article, writes thoughtfully and angrily about the stigma associated with being a single mother:

> The discourse around single parents, 90% of whom are women, is that they have shamelessly chosen their predicament. It seems that people don't break up because their relationships are no longer working or one partner is harming the other. No. Women, usually teenagers, the story goes, pick lone parenting and all the hardships it entails because they're guaranteed £72.40 a week and a council flat.[20]

Poverty and wellbeing

The above mention of single motherhood in the same sentence as welfare benefits leads us seamlessly onto the issue of single motherhood and poverty, and inescapably linked to this is the relationship between poverty and wellbeing.

When I became a single mother the fact that I was earning a good salary was important. I have always felt consciously grateful for being in a relatively secure position financially and know that this is not the experience of the majority of single mothers. On becoming a single mother, I did not, therefore, have worries about housing or having enough money for food and clothing etc. This also meant that I was able to use my salary to help me with the consequences of my new status as a single parent. Being able to leave the house and see friends for a few hours for an evening every now and then was important. It helped me to retain a sense of myself as an adult woman and stopped me from defining myself solely as a single mother and worker. I had enough money to afford to pay for babysitters periodically. I also had the support of good friends and neighbours who helped with childcare. Having a local community of support was a huge help, but, despite protestations from good friends, I tended to take up their offers of childcare as a last resort. This was not because I did not think that their offers were genuine, or that my children would not be safe or happy with them, but due to a strong sense of shame and a wish not to be perceived by others as a burden. It felt important that others could see that I could handle my single parent situation on my own and that I should not be dependent on anyone. Dorothy recalls the shame associated with having to ask for help:

> It always allowed me to 'dig deep' and carry on alone. With hindsight, I would do this differently – I would accept offers of help; I wouldn't feel the need to be fiercely independent and in control. I would also not judge other single mums if they needed to ask for help of any kind – but I judged (judge?!) myself.

Nelson carried out a study which involved interviewing, from a sociological perspective, four white, rural, American single mothers.[21] With an interest in exploring the concept of what Nelson describes as 'doing family', the paper acknowledges that single mothers' circumstances, coupled with often limited finances and other constraints, mean that single mothers often need other people. This challenges the traditional notion of family and those who single mothers see as, essentially, family, 'for help with daily survival. By virtue of doing so, they also have to make choices about who counts as family and they have to delineate appropriate activities for those they include.' Nelson suggests that this provides an opportunity for single mothers to operate a family structure outside that of the 'standard North American family'. However, her research suggests that the idea of a traditional family remains and is a powerful influence so that single mothers usually seek to recreate the standard nuclear family. She suggests that this may well be because the standard family unit provides order and predictability.

The majority of lone parents are consistently worse off financially than couple families, and single mothers are twice as likely as mothers in couple families to report poor health.[22] There is a well established link between poverty and the outcome for children. We know, for example, that growing up in poverty impacts negatively on children's health and their educational achievement. It has, therefore, been suggested that it might be that poverty is the significant factor in some of the difficulties experienced by some children of separated parents, rather than being bought up by a lone parent.[23] Indeed, the adverse effects of parental separation diminish or disappear entirely when financial income is controlled for.[24]

Linked to poverty is wellbeing – physical and mental. Brown and Moran found that single mothers are at greater risk of receiving a diagnosis of depression when compared with those living with a partner.[25] Their study compared a sample of inner-city single mothers living in Islington, North London, with a group of married or co-habiting mothers living in the same geographical area. They found that half of single mothers were among the bottom fifth of the population in income distribution compared with 22 per cent of married mothers. The risk of 'onset of depression' among single mothers was double that of the married sample and almost double among women in financial hardship. Such financial hardship was particularly common among single mothers.[26] The full-time employment of single mothers was seen in this study as related to financial hardship. A major reason for choosing to work full-time was to avoid poverty. Although most reported enjoying work, feelings of exhaustion were common, together with concern about possible neglect of their children. So the relationship between single motherhood and poverty is complex.

Brown and Moran's paper ends by acknowledging the extent to which the single mothers in their study remained aspirational in terms of achieving the best for their children despite their often very challenging circumstances:

> The lengthy interviews with the single mothers in this study left little doubt of the basic motive of the great majority to do well particularly by their children. We rarely sensed that they would not grasp opportunities to improve their lot if they arose. In this there must be hope of some way forward.[27]

Such findings challenge societal prejudice about how single mothers approach parenting and highlight the complexity of understanding the impact of being brought up by a single mother on children's lives and wellbeing.

Impact on children's lives

The popular view is that parental separation results, de facto, in emotionally and psychologically damaged children: '*Children from broken homes "twice as likely to be disruptive"*.'[28] Whilst being aware that I may be sensitive and selectively attentive to the reporting of such matters, I have noticed that news reports about those who have committed murder or manslaughter often include somewhere in their accounts the fact that the person who had committed the offence had come from a 'broken' family: '*Children from broken homes "nine times more likely to commit crimes"*.'[29] The implication here is that there is a causal link between having separated or divorced parents and being more likely to commit crimes. Such a claim requires closer examination of the evidence. Indeed, research strongly suggests that exposure to conflict between parents is the key mediating variable leading to emotional, psychological and behavioural difficulties in children rather than having separated parents *per se*.[30] This is summed up well by a report by Mooney and colleagues:

> A comparison between couple families experiencing high levels of conflict with single parents found that children fared less well in conflicted couple families, demonstrating that family functioning has a greater impact than family structure in contributing to child outcomes.[31]

The impact of family functioning and family structure on children is mediated by individual differences in children themselves. It has been suggested that the variation in children within the same family can be as great, if not greater, than the differences between children in different families.[32] This is supported by the knowledge that children differ in their levels of resilience and in their responses to stress.[33] However, there is evidence, too, that the quality of the relationship between parents and their children reduces as a result of separation.[34,35] Relevant to this is the impact of other factors that are associated with single motherhood, such as poverty and the psychological and emotional wellbeing of the single mother. These factors can also impact negatively on children's wellbeing.[36] Mooney and colleagues (2009) cite a study which found that the psychological wellbeing of the mother 'is more predictive of child outcomes than family structure'.[37]

An examination of the research evidence clearly demonstrates that quality of parenting plays a crucial role in the wellbeing of children, and this is the main predictor of children's wellbeing in both intact families and lone-parent families.[38,39] A report on parenting resilience notes that consistent and confident parenting by single mothers leads to children with fewer behavioural difficulties.[40] The parenting and attachment literature therefore shows that it is parenting style and the nature of the relationship between the parent and the child that are most crucial to ensuring children's wellbeing. This applies to lone parenting too.

There is clear evidence to suggest that there are some key factors that affect the wellbeing of children with a lone parent. Children fare better if their single mother has good mental health, if they have a positive relationship with their mother, and if the parenting style is emotionally warm and containing: 'Longitudinal research shows that good quality parent–child relationships and flexible arrangements can ameliorate many of the potentially negative effects of separation on children's wellbeing.'[41] This, of course, makes intuitive sense and also applies to two-parent families, but two-parent families tend to come under less societal scrutiny. This is further supported by research exploring protective factors that moderate the risks associated with being a child of separated or divorced parents. The study has found that these factors include better psychological adjustment, competent parenting and low parental conflict.[42]

On becoming a single parent due to bereavement

The experience of women who are single mothers due to the death of their partner is both similar and quite different to those who are single due to the ending of a relationship. The common assumption, however, is that a woman is a single mother due to separation or divorce. This is, perhaps, understandable given that only seven per cent of single parents have acquired this status as a consequence of the death of their partner.[43]

My colleague, Julie, the widowed mother of two young boys, observes that 'if one says that one is widowed, this usually brings about a mixed reaction of disbelief ("Did I hear you correctly?"), horror, sympathy and occasionally admiration. These reactions are particularly magnified if one is with young children at the time.'

Although there are commonalities faced by all single parents, acquiring this status due to the bereavement of a partner (particularly when the mother has young children or is pregnant, or both) brings about specific challenges with added layers of complexity. A qualitative study of five Canadian women, all single mothers who were under the age of 45 at the time of their husband's death, found themes in participants' experiences around loss, which included loss of companionship and loss of hopes and dreams.[44]

People often describe themselves as mourning the end of a relationship when separation occurs. However, a relationship ending through the death of a partner is different. When a partner dies, they are gone, in the physical sense, forever. Even if separated parents have no contact with one another, at least the possibility exists. Death is final. The surviving partner knows that they will never see their partner again and neither will their children. This requires the surviving parent to be able to manage not only their own grief but also that of their children. This is not a one-off event but a process that has no clear end in sight. Theoretically, we know that what is important in helping children cope with their grief is to keep alive the memory of their parent, always allowing for open, honest and developmentally appropriate conversation and expression of emotion. In doing so, however, on each occasion the surviving parent's own grief is triggered and needs to be managed. The age of a child when they lose a parent and the unique circumstances of the death all have an impact.

In losing their partner, the surviving single mother grieves for the experiences their children will never have, such as rough and tumble play with their father, playing football with their father in the park/back garden, and the proud father walking his daughter down the aisle. Lowe and McClement found a key theme related to loss of family relationships and activities.[45] In the case of heterosexual couples, the surviving parent will be acutely aware of the loss of a primary gender role model (depending upon which parent has died) and will have a desire to try to create that for their child/children where possible.

The UK national charity Widowed and Young (WAY) was founded in 1997.[46] WAY recognises the specific support required for young widows and widowers. WAY is a peer-to-peer support network run by, and for, men and women who were aged 50 or under when their partner died. Local support networks are located throughout the UK. WAY talks about young widows/widowers with children as being 'double parents'. This term seems to encapsulate the essence of being widowed with children. All responsibility lies with the surviving parent. There is no other parent to share the load, to make decisions with, to pick up a sick child from school, to look after the children whilst the other parent has some time for themselves etc. Importantly, in addition, the surviving parent feels a responsibility to try to be both mother and father, both practically and emotionally. Being a double parent can be emotionally and physically exhausting, and Lowe and McClement highlighted this as a key finding of their study: 'The complexity of children's needs becomes clearer when one is forced to be responsible for everything alone.'[47] Another study of women who are widows provides further evidence for this, having found that women missed their partner's role in discipline and decision-making and struggled with taking on the roles of both mother and father.[48]

Dorothy reflects on the huge sense of responsibility she feels as a single mother and the impact this has:

> The feeling of overwhelming responsibility is one of the hardest, scariest things. I joke that I'm the first and last line of defence for my children against the world. It's a sobering thought. It's impacted on my decisions to undertake opportunities.

Widowed parents, like other single parents, can at times feel envy towards – and different in comparison to – families where there are two parents at home. In addition, they may also feel different to other single parents – they may no longer be with their partner but at least their ex-partner and mother/father of their child/children is still alive. Young widows/widowers can feel isolated from both married/cohabiting couples and other single parents. Perhaps that is why having the support of an organisation such as WAY can be so important. Another extremely important aspect of such a group is that children get to meet and form friendships with other children who have also lost a parent due to bereavement, thereby hopefully addressing to some extent their own sense of difference and potential isolation.

As challenging as being a widowed parent can be, there are positives. First, the surviving parent has total autonomy over their decisions and there are no arguments over differing parental practices. This can be a difficult path to navigate but to do so can provide a real sense of achievement and competence. This highlights the resilience of the surviving parent and is a reminder to them of the important concept of being a 'good enough parent'.[49] This helps to foster compassion in oneself and acts as a reminder that what is ultimately important for children is having a secure base from which a secure attachment can develop and thrive. Working parents provide a role model for their children, and being a 'double parent' provides an example of non-stereotypical gender roles.

On reflecting on being a double parent due to the death of her husband, Julie sums all of this up succinctly:

> My children might be late for school (sometimes), not had time to brush their hair (often), forgotten their PE kit, homework (again) but they are well behaved (most of the time!), have good friendships, are happy, healthy and we experience together a very strong bond and secure attachment.

Parenting as teamwork

When Julie first talked to me about being a 'double parent' this made me stop and think about what this meant. This clearly applies particularly to lone parents who are single due to the death of their partner – the other parent no longer exists so the surviving parent is under pressure to be a double parent. However, mothers who are single through divorce or separation may also feel that they are required to be a double parent. For some, this will be because their child or children are estranged from their father. Others may feel that they are a double parent despite the fact that their child or children have contact with their father. Indeed, there are days when I feel like I am the same person playing numerous different roles – just like an actor who plays several different characters in a farce. I notice, in the daily narratives of couples' lives, themes of teamwork and of a sharing of roles. A friend may talk about how she did the food shopping and cooking at the weekend while her partner helped the children to do their homework and then did some gardening. A colleague, on a Monday morning, talks about going out with friends on the previous Saturday night, leaving her husband to collect their son from a party. It is hard, as a single mother, not to envy this apparently well-oiled machine of effective team work, of partnership in parenting.

My father died during the period of time that I have been writing this chapter. He lived about 200 miles from me, so during his final few weeks I found myself doing my usual full-time job Monday to Friday and then travelling to be with him at the weekends. This brought into sharp focus some of the many consequences of single motherhood. Interwoven with complex feelings about the imminent death of my father was a powerful sense of not being present enough for my children. This was compounded by the knowledge that my daughters were both upset and worried about their grandfather's ill health and the likelihood of his imminent death. The decision to leave them the day after my father died, in order to be with family members to mourn together and plan the funeral, felt particularly difficult. In six years of being a single mother I have often wished to have the ability to be in two places at once.

Dorothy describes her sadness at not being able to share the parenting good times:

> Even the 'good times' can be heart-breaking as there is no one to share them with, to also revel in your pride in your kids or what they may have achieved. Part of me always used to dread the 'happy times', such as Christmas, as they are holidays and events that can magnify the 'smallness' of our family. I coped by overcompensating with enthusiasm and jolliness to hopefully create a strong sense of togetherness and family. I hope it worked and my two girls look back at these childhood times with happiness. Time will tell.

Attachment

The concept of attachment requires some exploration in relation to single motherhood and the relationship between single mothers and their children. Bowlby's theory of attachment primarily describes the enduring emotional bond that forms between infants and their primary caregivers.[50] Bowlby was inspired by evolutionary theory and viewed attachment as an evolutionary mechanism. Attachment is characterised by an individual wanting to be in close contact with their attachment figure and experiencing involuntary separation from them as highly distressing. The attachment figure is sought out to provide comfort, support and protection at times of distress, and is depended upon as a 'secure base' from which the individual can freely explore the world. Based on the development of early attachment bonds formed between infants and their primary caregivers, infants go on to develop a unique set of expectations or mental representations of themselves and others in attachment relationships.[51]

Bowlby's initial focus was on how attachment theory explained what was happening in the relationship between infants and their primary caregivers. However, he went on to describe how attachment representations influence the formation of relationships in adulthood.[52] Bowlby argued that internal working models of self and others form a template for future relationships.

So, what can attachment theory tell us about the impact of lone parenting on children's emotional wellbeing and ability to form secure relationships? Miljkovitch, Danet and Bernier have carried out a study to examine child attachment in the context of single parenthood – both maternal and paternal – and to investigate 'intergenerational transmission of attachment' in single-parent–child dyads compared with two-parent families.[53] The authors' aim was specifically to explore this in single parent dyads, as previous research in the area had largely been studied in intact families. Miljkovitch and colleagues argue that research into attachment in single-parent families is unclear due to the number of confounding variables that obscure the findings.[54] For example, it is understood that insecure attachment occurs at a higher rate when in conjunction with negative life events. So what may be perceived and presented as a clear research finding – that children are less securely attached to their mothers in single-parent families – is actually much more complicated. Insecure and/or disorganised attachment results from marital conflict, and not all relationships will end due to marital conflict, so children may develop insecure attachments within two-parent families.[55]

Miljkovitch and colleagues explored parent and child attachment in 50 married couples and 43 single parents (22 mothers and 21 fathers) of children aged between three and six years. They administered the Adult Attachment Interview and the Attachment Story Completion Task to measure child and adult attachment representations.[56] The researchers found that children's attachment representations differed according to family structure. Those children raised solely by their fathers had higher disorganisation scores than those raised solely by their mothers. The study's authors conclude that, 'Taken together, these findings suggest that single parenthood per se is not linked to more insecure or disorganized child attachment representations. However, when the father is the only caregiver, children exhibit more disorganised representations.'[57] The authors acknowledge that this finding could be due to a number of different factors. They found a decrease in intergenerational transmission of secure attachment in single mothers. They suggest that this is most likely to be caused by the changes in circumstances for the single mother, leading to increase in financial hardship, the trauma due to the breakup of their relationship, and the fact that being solely responsible could result in a reduction in maternal sensitivity and responsiveness which in turn may reduce the transmission of attachment security. Given that attachment is a much-researched concept, it would seem that there is a need for further exploration of the impact of lone parenting on attachment in a way that teases out and identifies the relevant factors – rather than making an assumption of a simple causal link between lone parenting and forms of insecure attachment.

Resilience

Formal definitions of resilience vary but key to any definition is a capacity to deal with severe adversity.[58] The concept of resilience is usually defined as doing well or better than expected under difficult circumstances. There has been considerable interest in exploring the concept of resilience in numerous contexts in recent years – from those factors that promote resilience following childhood sexual abuse, to psychological resilience in sport and exploring resilience in the context of a period of societal austerity.[59,60,61] Much of the focus has been on what enables resilience in people and why some prove to be more resilient in response to adverse life events and experiences. This is pertinent to an understanding of the impact of separation/divorce on children and to an understanding of why some children fare better than others.

Hsieh and Leung have explored what enables resilience in 291 Taiwanese teenagers (with a mean age of 13 years) of divorced parents.[62] A central finding of this study was that positive family functioning within the divorced families – such that the family functioned in ways that were coherent, harmonious and supportive – enabled the young person to adjust better to their parents' divorce and new circumstances. Similar findings were also reported by Greef, Vansteenwegen and DeMot in a study of 68 Belgian divorced families.[63]

Levine, in a study of 15 single mothers of disabled children, aimed to identify the individual, family, social and environmental factors that help to enable resilience in this population. Her study identified four main themes that accounted for the resilience in the mothers that were interviewed. One of these is described by Levine as the participants having developed a view of their position as single mothers that noticed and celebrated their 'mother-presence' which replaced father absence. Levine notes that these women preferred their lone-parent status over staying in unsatisfying relationships.[64]

What seems clear is that being a child of separated or divorced parents *per se* does not automatically lead to adverse outcomes; a number of factors mediate the impact of parental separation on children. Indeed, children who grow up in families with two parents are also at risk of adverse outcomes, particularly if they experience significant parental conflict or if their parents have low financial incomes. It is nevertheless clear that single motherhood still carries a stigma, and that some of the research findings are negative with regards to the wellbeing of single mothers and the impact on children of being brought up by a single mother. However, within the research literature, as well as the media, there is also much written that is positive – this particularly celebrates the strength of single mothers and notices much evidence of coping and resilience in this group. Brown and Moran note:

> One hazard of discussing the experiences of a social category such as single mother is presenting an essentially bleak picture, while being aware of inspiring instances of effective coping ... feelings of role success and competence in terms of a sense of doing well with regard to motherhood, employment, intimacy in sexual relationships and social contacts with friends and relatives was common.[65]

Dorothy describes how she and her daughters have become more resilient together:

> Now my girls are older ... I'm now at a stage where I feel pride in the three of us – what we have managed, what we have done together. We describe ourselves as 'a three-legged stool' – each of us is a leg and when we are together and well we are sturdy and strong!

The positives of single motherhood

When I first became a single mother I was acutely conscious of seeming something other and different to the majority of adults/parents whom I knew – I was a single mother and, of course, a single woman. Most adults live their lives in partnerships. I worried about the emotional impact on my children of having separated parents, and envied those couples I knew whose relationships seemed secure and happy. I have always said that I would not have chosen to be a single mother nor for my children to have separated parents. However, six years on I am much more aware of some of the positives of my situation. Echoing Julie's comments earlier in this chapter, I do not have to negotiate approaches to parenting with a partner nor argue about who is responsible for domestic chores and childcare – it is all my sole responsibility. I have also become aware that my previous tendency to idealise those in long-term relationships is misplaced. Many long-term couple relationships are troubled and it could be argued that some children of parents who are together but unhappy experience more worry and unhappiness than those whose parents are separated and where the status of their parents' relationship is clear. I find myself surprised by friends occasionally saying that they envy my lifestyle – they see that I have freedoms in certain ways that they do not.

Without doubt, single motherhood comes with a host of challenges. It can be lonely and very hard work, and, as discussed here, it is still seen by society as largely negative. However, the research findings show that apparently simple causal links are misplaced and the picture is more complex than the media would lead us to believe. Some key ingredients need to be present for children to have a happy, safe and fulfilled life, and these ingredients are not exclusively found in two-parent families.

It seems apt, then, to end this chapter with a quote from J.K. Rowling, who describes her pride at navigating a period in her life as a single mother and articulates some of the positives:

> I would say to any single parent currently feeling the weight of stereotype or stigmatization that I am prouder of my years as a single mother than of any other part of my life. Yes, I got off benefits and wrote the first four *Harry Potter* books as a single mother, but nothing makes me prouder than what Jessica told me recently about the first five years of her life: 'I never knew we were poor. I just remember being happy.'[66]

Acknowledgements

Many thanks go to Julie Robinson for contributing the section in this chapter on becoming a single parent due to bereavement. My thanks also go to Julie, as well as Jane Thorpe and Dorothy Frizelle, for sharing their experiences as single mothers with me, for their comments on a draft of this chapter, and for allowing me to use their words.

Endnotes

1. Paton, G. (2010). Children in single parent families 'worse behaved'. Available at http://www.telegraph.co.uk/education/educationnews/8064435/Children-in-single-parent-families-worse-behaved.html (retrieved 18 March 2015).
2. Waterlow, L. (2014). The single mother of eight children planning a lavish Christmas – all funded by benefits worth £2,200 a MONTH. Available at http://www.dailymail.co.uk/femail/article-2877774/The-single-mother-eight-children-planning-lavish-Christmas-funded-benefits-worth-2-200-MONTH.html (retrieved 18 March 2015).
3. Beckford, M. (2008). Children in single-parent families more likely to suffer emotional problems, report finds. Available at http://www.telegraph.co.uk/news/politics/3235650/Children-in-single-parent-families-more-likely-to-suffer-emotional-problems-report-finds.html (retrieved 18 March 2015).

4. Sherine, A. (2014) Being a single parent is no picnic. Available at http://www.theguardian.com/lifeandstyle/2014/jan/04/single-parent-no-picnic-low-income-children (retrieved 18 March 2015).
5. Office for National Statistics (2012). *Families and Households, 2012.* Available at http://www.ons.gov.uk/ons/rel/family-demography/families-and-households/2012/stb-families-households.html (retrieved 21 April 2015).
6. Mooney, A., Oliver, C. & Smith, M. (2009). *Impact of Family Breakdown on Children's Well-being: Evidence review.* London: Department for Children, Schools and Families.
7. Jadva, V., Badger, S., Morrissette, M. & Golombok, S. (2009). 'Mom by choice, single by life's circumstance...': Findings from a large scale survey of the experiences of single mothers by choice. *Human Fertility, 12*, 175–184.
8. Office for National Statistics (2012). *Families and Households, 2012.* Available at http://www.ons.gov.uk/ons/rel/family-demography/families-and-households/2012/stb-families-households.html (retrieved 21 April 2015).
9. Ibid.
10. Wade, T. J., Veldhuizen, S. & Cairney, J. (2011). Prevalence of psychiatric disorder in lone fathers and mothers: Examining the intersection of gender and family structure on mental health. *Canadian Journal of Psychiatry, 56*, 567–573.
11. Ibid.
12. United States Census Bureau (2012). Family groups with children under 18 years old by race and Hispanic origin: 1990 to 2012. Available at http://www.census.gov/prod/cen2010/briefs/c2010br-14.pdf (retrieved 18 March 2015).
13. INSEE (2012). Tableaux de l'économie française. Available at http://www.insee.fr/fr/ffc/tef/tef2012/tef2012.pdf (retrieved 18 March 2015).
14. Gingerbread (n.d.). Statistics. Available at http://www.gingerbread.org.uk/content/365/statistics (retrieved 18 March 2015).
15. Levine, K. (2009). Resilience as authoritative knowledge: The experiences of single mothers of children with disabilities. *Journal of the Association for Research on Mothering, 10*, 133–145.
16. Gingerbread (2014). Stigma alive and well in 2014, say three in four single parents. Available at http://www.gingerbread.org.uk/news/248/mothers-day-stigma (retrieved 18 March 2015).
17. Rowling, J. K. (n.d.). I am prouder of my years as a single mother than of any other part of my life. Available at http://www.gingerbread.org.uk/content/1901/J-K-Rowling (retrieved 18 March 2015).
18. Ibid.
19. Gingerbread (n.d.). Statistics. Available at http://www.gingerbread.org.uk/content/365/statistics (retrieved 18 March 2015).
20. Okolosie, L. (2014). Hooray for single mothers – and Gillian Wearing's celebration of them. Available at http://www.theguardian.com/commentisfree/2014/oct/31/single-mothers-gillian-wearing-traditional-family-statue-birmingham (retrieved 18 March 2015).
21. Nelson, M. (2006). Single mothers 'do' family. *Journal of Marriage and Family, 68*, 781–795.
22. Lyon, N. Barnes, M. & Sweiry, D. (2006). *Families with Children in Britain: Findings from the 2004 Families and Children Study (FACS)* (DWP Research Report No. 340). Leeds: Corporate Document Services.
23. Mooney, A., Oliver, C. & Smith, M. (2009). *Impact of Family Breakdown on Children's Well-being: Evidence review.* London: Department for Children, Schools and Families.
24. Mackay, R. (2005). The impact of family structure and family change on child outcomes: A personal reading of the research literature. *Social Policy Journal of New Zealand, 24*, 111–133.

25. Brown, G. & Moran, P. (1997). Single mothers, poverty and depression. *Psychological Medicine, 27,* 21–33.
26. Ibid.
27. Ibid.
28. Clark, L. (2010). Children from broken homes twice as likely to be disruptive. Available at http://www.dailymail.co.uk/news/article-1320648/Children-broken-homes-twice-likely-disruptive.html (retrieved 18 March 2015).
29. Bloxham, A. (2010). Children from broken homes 'nine times more likely to commit crimes'. Available at http://www.telegraph.co.uk/news/politics/8109184/Children-from-broken-homes-nine-times-more-likely-to-commit-crimes.html (retrieved 18 March 2015).
30. Mooney, A., Oliver, C. & Smith, M. (2009). *Impact of Family Breakdown on Children's Well-being: Evidence review.* London: Department for Children, Schools and Families.
31. Ibid.
32. O'Connor, T. G., Dunn, J., Jenkins, J.M., Pickering, K. & Rasbash, J. (2001). Family settings and children's adjustment: Differential adjustment within and across families. *British Journal of Psychiatry, 179,* 110–115.
33. Hetherington, E. M. & Stanley-Hagan, M. (1999). The adjustment of children with divorced parents: A risk and resiliency perspective. *Journal of Child Psychology and Psychiatry, 40,* 129–140.
34. Emery, R. E. (1982). Interparental conflict and the children of discord and divorce. *Psychological Bulletin, 92,* 310–330.
35. Emery, R. E. (1994). *Renegotiating Family Relationships: Divorce, child custody and mediation.* New York: Guilford Press.
36. Bainham, A., Lindley, B., Richards, M. & Trinder, L. (Eds) (2003). *Children and Their Families: Contact rights and welfare.* Oxford: Hart.
37. Smith, M. (2004). Parental mental health: Disruptions to parenting and outcomes for children. *Child and Family Social Work, 9,* 3–11. Cited in Mooney, A. et al., 2009. See note 30.
38. Amato, P. R. (2005). The impact of family formation change on the cognitive, social and emotional well-being of the next generation. *The Future of Children, 15,* 75–96.
39. Dunn, J. (2005). Daddy doesn't live here anymore. *The Psychologist, 18,* 28–31.
40. Hill, M., Stafford, A., Seaman, P., Ross, N. & Daniel, B. (2007). *Parenting and Resilience.* York: Joseph Rowntree Foundation.
41. Neale, G. & Flowerdew, J. (2007). New structure, new agency: The dynamics of child–parent relationships after divorce. *International Journal of Children's Rights, 51,* 25–42. Cited in Mooney, A. et al., 2009. See note 30.
42. Kelly, J. B. & Emery, R. E. (2003). Children's adjustment following divorce: Risk and resilience perspectives. *Family Relations, 52,* 352–362.
43. Gingerbread (n.d.). Consultation responses – welfare and benefits. Available at http://www.gingerbread.org.uk/content/664/Consultation-responses---benefits (retrieved 18 March 2015).
44. Lowe, M. E. & McClement, S. E. (2010). Spousal bereavement: The lived experience of young Canadian widows. *OMEGA, 62,* 127–148.
45. Ibid.
46. See WAY – Widowed & Young: https://www.widowedandyoung.org.uk/ (retrieved 18 March 2015).
47. See note 44.
48. Lopata, H. Z. (1996). *Current Widowhood.* New York: Elsevier.
49. Winnicott, D. W. (1973). *The Child, the Family and the Outside World.* Harmondsworth: Penguin, p. 173.

50. Bowlby, J. (1969). *Attachment and Loss: Volume 1: Attachment*. New York: Basic Books.
51. Ibid.
52. Bowlby, J. (1979). *The Making and Breaking of Affectional Bonds*. London: Tavistock.
53. Miljkovitch, R., Danet, M. & Bernier, A. (2012). Intergenerational transmission of attachment representations in the context of single parenthood in France. *Journal of Family Psychology, 26,* 784–792.
54. Ibid.
55. Finger, B., Hans, S. L., Berstein, V. J. & Cox, S. M. (2009). Parent relationship quality and infant-mother attachment. *Attachment & Human Development, 11,* 285–306.
56. See note 53.
57. Ibid.
58. Hill, M., Stafford, A., Seaman, P., Ross, N. & Daniel, B. (2007). *Parenting and Resilience*. York: Joseph Rowntree Foundation.
59. Marriott, C., Hamilton-Giachritsis, C. & Harrop, C. (2014). Factors promoting resilience following childhood sexual abuse: A structured, narrative review of the literature. *Child Abuse Review, 23,* 17–34.
60. Galli, N. & Gonzalez, S. P. (2014). Psychological resilience in sport: A review of the literature and implications for research and practice. *International Journal of Sport and Exercise Psychology* [online]. Available at http://www.tandfonline.com/doi/full/10.1080/1612197X.2014.946947#abstract (retrieved 22 April 2015).
61. Robertson, I. & Cooper, C. (2013). Resilience (editorial). *Stress and Health, 29,* 175–176.
62. Hsieh, M.-O. & Leung, P. (2009). Protective factors for adolescents among divorced single-parent families from Taiwan. *Social Work in Health Care, 48,* 298–320.
63. Greef, A.P., Vansteenwegen, A. & DeMot, L. (2006). Resiliency in divorced families. *Social Work in Mental Health, 4,* 67–81.
64. Levine, K. (2009). Resilience as authoritative knowledge: The experiences of single mothers of children with disabilities. *Journal of the Association for Research on Mothering, 10,* 133–145.
65. Brown, G. & Moran, P. (1997). Single mothers, poverty and depression. *Psychological Medicine, 27,* 21–33.
66. See note 17.

Chapter 6
Considering the relationship between vulnerability and child sexual exploitation

Adele Gladman

This chapter looks at the issues of vulnerability in relation to child sexual exploitation. Is vulnerability something that is created by being involved or exposed to CSE? Is it present in the young person at the outset and playing a role in their involvement? In some cases, is it both? If it is something that leads to the young person being targeted and involved then perhaps the most crucial questions of all are, what causes the vulnerability in the first place, and can practitioners work proactively by recognising it, addressing it, and in doing so prevent harm to children?

In this chapter I will consider traditional perceptions of vulnerability; the emergence of a new type of vulnerability to CSE; professional responses and created vulnerability; perceptions of CSE as a child protection issue; and ways forward.[1]

What is child sexual exploitation?

CSE is child abuse. Government guidance describes it as follows:

> The sexual exploitation of children and young people under 18 involves exploitative situations, contexts and relationships where young people (or a third person or persons) receive something (e.g. food, accommodation, drugs, alcohol, cigarettes, affections, gifts, money) as a result of them performing, and/or another or others performing on them, sexual activities.
>
> Child sexual exploitation can occur through the use of technology without the child's immediate recognition; for example being persuaded to post sexual images on the internet/mobile phones without immediate payment or gain.

> In all cases those exploiting the child/young person have power over them by virtue of their age, gender, intellect, physical strength and/or economic or other resources.
>
> Violence, coercion and intimidations are common, involvement in exploitative relationships being characterised in the main by the child's or young person's limited availability of choice resulting from their social/economic and/or emotional vulnerability.[2]

I first became interested in the above questions and the relationship between vulnerability and CSE when working on a Home Office-funded research and development pilot that ran in Rotherham, South Yorkshire, from 2000 to 2002. At that time there were growing concerns about young women who were becoming involved in CSE in Rotherham.[3,4] A specialist project, the Risky Business project, had been established within the Youth Service to better understand these young people's experiences and offer them support. By the time the Home Office-funded pilot began, a considerable number of young people were accessing the project. In this chapter I have drawn on my experiences of working with those young women, and other young women with whom I have worked since. The cases I cite are composite and not identifiable to any individual or family, but the details are all true.[5] I have deliberately not quoted from any research or academic work because I want the experiences of these young women to speak for themselves and not become obscured by statistical and academic analysis.

Traditional views of vulnerability

When I first started working with young women who were believed to be involved in CSE, I identified that a significant number had experiences in their lives that may have resulted in them being considered vulnerable by the services working with them. Some had been abused – often by parents, family members, carers, or by others known and trusted by them. Others had been neglected through poor parenting or exposure to parental substance misuse. Some had parents who were recipients of mental health or learning disability services. Some had experienced domestic violence and abuse, or repeated relationship breakdown. Some had repeated experiences of their mother forming new relationships and had been required to regard and address each new adult male partner as their father. It was apparent that, because of these factors, some of the young women known to the project were extremely vulnerable prior to becoming involved in CSE. They were often isolated and unhappy, had low self-esteem or confidence, were bullied at school, and had no concept of what a healthy relationship was. Many of them were already known to statutory services as a result of concerns being raised by education or other services.

Those children who had been neglected and emotionally abused in particular seemed to be desperately seeking relationships of any kind – validation that they meant something to someone, that someone valued them as a human being and cared for them, that they were not invisible to the world.

This type of vulnerability can be explored through T's story. T had experienced severe emotional and sexual abuse from a young age. By the time T was removed into local authority care at the age of 10, she had been sexually abused by multiple perpetrators, had been severely neglected for most of her life, was developmentally behind her peers, and was also estranged from them in terms of her social development and friendships. In summary, T was a damaged, lonely and isolated child.

T's first foster placement broke down almost immediately as a result of her behaviour. T missed her family and wanted to return home. She did not understand why she had been removed from her family. When T was placed in a residential home and another resident showed an interest in her, T was probably both flattered and grateful. When the other girl suggested that they run away for 'a bit of fun', T was more than happy to go. When T was introduced by her new-found friend to a man in his twenties, and this man showed an interest in her and paid her compliments, T wanted to see him again.

By the time the project became involved, T believed that she was in love with this man and he with her. The abuse she was experiencing was prolific, but nothing was too much to give to the man who told her that she was pretty, that he loved her; the man who kissed and cuddled her and made her feel special – before passing her on to have sex with a number of other adult males; the man who, in effect, had become her abuser in place of the father she missed so much, and who she wasn't allowed to see.

There are several elements to T's story:

- Her abuse from an early age and abuse that became so regular that it was the norm – part of her routine, part of day-to-day life for an unloved and uncared-for little girl, who did not know that other children did not live like this.

- The absence of love and affection, or any acknowledgement of her needs, except when she was fulfilling someone else's.
- The invisibility surrounding her abuse: issues of neglect and developmental delay would have undoubtedly been picked up by the school she attended and perhaps reported to social care, but the reality of her life did not become known until years later, when she was finally removed from the family home and placed into the care of the local authority.
- The isolation from her peers: from the start T was different. She was a little girl with a big secret. Almost certainly she would have had very little in common with her peers because of her dysfunctional home life and distorted relationship with her father and other adults. Her family was unlikely to have encouraged her to form friendships with her peers and, given the family's reputation in the community, not many other families would have encouraged their daughters to be friends with T.
- The isolation from her community: the family had a reputation, as stated above. But no one took any action to protect this little girl or raise concerns about her with social care or the police. It is easy to see how, in these circumstances, children like T feel invisible to the world, and how easy it is for abusers to control and manipulate them.
- Once T was taken into care, attempts were made to ascertain her wishes and feelings. It is accepted that great care has to be taken when talking to young people about abuse they have experienced, particularly at the hands of someone that they loved and trusted. In T's case, however, the issues were discussed so diplomatically and carefully that T did not understand why she had been removed from the family home and why she was not able to see her family. T did not see herself as a victim of abuse. She did not understand why her foster carer's husband and other male members of the family had been advised by social care not to be left alone with her. She was experiencing bereavement and loss, and was not receiving any therapeutic intervention to help her understand and cope with this. She also did not have a single person to whom she could talk honestly and frankly about her life. With the benefit of hindsight, the foster placement

was almost certain to break down from the moment that T arrived.

- T was placed in a residential setting as it was felt that she might settle better and benefit more from living with some of her peers. None of the vulnerability factors identified were addressed. The home was regarded as a place of safety, somewhere where T could live and be cared for while her abuse was investigated, her needs assessed, and a decision made about her long-term care. What might happen to T in the interim, in a placement where there were already concerns about adult males collecting vulnerable young women by car, was apparently not considered; at the very least it was not acted on.

Considering T's case, it was possible to conclude that all of these issues of vulnerability led to three things: first, a young girl desperate for love, attention and affection; second, an opportunity for her vulnerability to be noticed and used to target, groom, abuse and control her; third, T's absolute loyalty to those who provided her with 'love', even if this was at a terrible cost. T's relationship with her abusers continued until she was no longer of interest to them. The end result was a child who blamed herself for some perceived wrongdoing, and was even more vulnerable and desperate than she had been when she first arrived in care.

Disability and vulnerability

While T's family history was extreme in its abuse, initially most of the young women known to the Risky Business project appeared to have some identifiable vulnerability, albeit of different types and differing levels.

Disability played a significant role in many cases. For C, it was why she was targeted in the first place. She was 16 years old and had been placed in foster care as a result of neglect in the family home and her parents' inability or unwillingness to care for her. C's functioning was variable; at some levels she was like a child of six, and this isolated her from girls of her age. She was friendly and trusting of those who showed an interest in her, and her vulnerability was obvious to any observer.

She also did not understand much about sexual activity because those around her had not talked to her about it. This was partly the result of an assessment by those working with and caring for her that she was like a little girl, so they treated her like a child who had no sexual feelings or interest. The correct approach would have been to recognise that physically she was a young adult and would have been experiencing feelings that are a natural part of adolescence. The failure to acknowledge C's adolescent development resulted in a belief that to speak to her about healthy relationships and sex would be inappropriate.

C's lack of awareness, combined with her easy-going, friendly and trusting nature, were spotted by a group of perpetrators and enabled them to approach and groom her. They were able to persuade her to go with them without resistance. They were able to give her alcohol and drugs because that was something else that she knew nothing about and they could persuade her it was 'just a bit of fun'. C was keen to please and fit in with her new friends. Over a period of time they were able to normalise sexual touching, to persuade C to keep secrets from her carers, and to come to them of her own volition.

Gradually, over time, they were able to abuse her by more than touching, and this often involved several acts of abuse by several different abusers. They were able to keep her for increasing amounts of time, in the knowledge that, even though C did not like what they were doing to her, she was not likely to put up resistance or tell anyone about it. Even if she did tell anyone, she was unlikely to be believed. Children with intellectual disabilities have rarely appeared as witnesses in cases at Crown Court, and obtaining coherent and persuasive evidence from them is often a time-consuming and difficult task.

When the abuse was detected the police became involved and identified several challenges that they argued prevented them from taking action against her abusers. One was C's age, even though she clearly lacked the requisite capacity to give free and informed consent to sexual intercourse. Another was that C was unable to name many of her abusers, although she was able to identify the address where she was being abused. As a result, her abuse was subject to further enquiries by the police. One of the many frustrating things about C's case was that there was often DNA evidence present on and in C's body after she had been abused. In other words, there was no need to rely entirely on C's account of what was happening to her and there were opportunities to investigate this further that were never explored. This was because C's abuse was regarded entirely as a consensual relationship, even though she did not have the capacity to give such consent.

As a result of this decision, C was left to continue being abused. From C's point of view, this reinforced the notion that her 'friends' were doing nothing wrong. I shall return to the issue of professional responses and increased vulnerability later in this chapter.

D is a different example of how disability created a vulnerability that was identified and used by an abuser. D suffered a serious injury in an accident and, after a long spell in hospital, returned to school needing to use a wheelchair. Her long absence from school meant she had fallen behind educationally and, by the time she returned, her friends had moved on, leaving her socially isolated too. She struggled to establish new friendships. Her isolation from her peers did not go unnoticed by an abuser 'window shopping' near the school. D was introduced to her abuser the same week by another pupil at her school, who was being abused by this man.

The tactics used to ensnare D drew directly on her circumstances – she was presented with a group of 'friends' who encouraged her to feel entitled to 'kick back', relax and have fun. Meeting an attractive older male who was attracted to her and who didn't care about the wheelchair was something that D had thought would never be possible.

When the abuse started D still believed that her abuser was her friend and lover. Later, when she began to question the relationship, threats and acts of severe violence towards her and her family were used to control her. D was forced to witness horrific acts of abuse on other young women. She felt compelled to protect her family and believed that the threats were real and would be carried out unless she complied. D's abuse continued well into her adult life.

'Looked after' children

A different vulnerability was identified in the young women who were looked after by the local authority. Whether they were accommodated through parental agreement or through an order of the court, they were in care because they had often experienced severe abuse and neglect and were considered to be at significant risk of harm if they remained living at home. The decision to remove children into care is never taken lightly by a local authority. An observation that I made throughout my years in practice, however, was that there was often a lot of activity and involvement by a range of different professionals in the months leading up to the young person being removed from home. But once a decision was made to accommodate the young person, this activity often dissipated, leaving just a handful of services trying to address numerous and complex needs, issues and risks, against ever-increasing workloads and ever-decreasing budgets.

Additionally, young people coming into the care system have often experienced significant trauma. They are rarely referred to any therapeutic services until indicators of this trauma begin to appear – through them going missing, for example, or behavioural clues.

Both when I was in Rotherham and since, I have encountered cases where young people in the care of the local authority and living in residential homes were targeted by abusers involved in CSE. Sometimes this would be facilitated by other young people who were living there and already involved with abusive adults. Sometimes young people were encouraged to go out with and go missing with their peers; they were introduced to a new set of 'friends' who eventually either passed them to other adult males or abused them themselves. The evidence collected during the Rotherham pilot suggested that abusers knew what they could get away with – for example, whether they could park outside and collect young people from a home; whether a home had CCTV; which homes had more proactive and protective staff; whether they could have associations with a group of residents or get away with just an individual relationship; what time young people had to be returned in order for them to avoid being reported as missing; and the extent of workers' powers to physically restrain or stop a young person from having contact with an abuser or leaving the home. Sometimes the young people had got to know the legalities and procedures – that residential workers could not use force to stop them leaving the home; that the police could not take action without the young person making a complaint, especially if they said that they were 'consenting' to their relationship; that they had the right to refuse to be medically examined. One child of 14 explained to me that she was 'Gillick competent' and that this meant she could do what she wanted.[6]

On more than one occasion I noted a pattern in which a previously good relationship and attachment to a parent or carer broke down, often accompanied by an allegation of abuse (usually physical) made by the young person against their carer. The young person would then ask to be placed into institutional care. In more than one case, either I or the project worker was later told by the young person that their abuser had suggested they use this tactic to get them away from the protection of carers and parents and into a setting where they believed the young person would be more accessible to them.

Emerging vulnerabilities in relation to CSE

In this chapter I have considered several different types of vulnerability that were a contributing factor to the young person becoming involved in CSE. It is important, however, to consider another group. During the course of the Rotherham pilot I started to identify a significant number of young people who did not meet the expected profile of vulnerability. These young women were not abused or neglected and did not come from dysfunctional families. The young people accessing the Risky Business project came from a variety of backgrounds and circumstances and many of them were still living with loving and caring families. These young women were also not considered troubled young people. This led me to ask, what was it that led to them becoming involved in CSE?

I identified a number of different circumstances that had created vulnerabilities in these young women or opportunities to target them. One frequent factor was the young person's experiences at school. Some young women were experiencing challenges that would not be uncommon for adolescents – they felt that they did not belong or were having difficulties in making and maintaining friendships. Some missed their friends from primary schools, who had gone on to other secondary schools. Others simply struggled with the transition from the primary to secondary setting. Some young people were having difficulties with educational attainment and achievement, which was distressing them and made them feel different from their peer group. Some were experiencing bullying at school.

Other young women were simply unhappy. In some cases this was because they were not getting on with parents or siblings; because their parents were having relationship difficulties or had separated; or because a close family member had died. S's case shows how this created a different type of vulnerability that ultimately led to an involvement in CSE.

S was 15 and from a close and loving family. Then her mother suddenly died. Her father was devastated and, while he tried his best to manage and support his daughter, he could not bear to talk about S's mother. He removed all photographs of her in the family home. S could see that her father was consumed by grief. He seemed unable to function and she observed him breaking down on a daily basis. The extent of his grief meant S felt totally unable to grieve for her mother herself or to talk to him about how she was feeling, in case she made his grief worse. Family members and friends told her that they understood how difficult it must be for her but that it was her job to care for her father now. They intimated, at least from S's perspective, that her father's grief must be greater (and therefore more important) than her own. S began to feel resentful of this burden that she did not ask for and did not want. She felt that no one else could possibly understand what she was going through. She began avoiding the family home as much as possible.

Eventually, on one occasion when she had gone missing from home, she was approached by an apparently kind and concerned member of the public. And there began the grooming process that would eventually lead to her being sexually exploited over a lengthy period of time. Her abuse would irreparably change her relationship with her family and her future life.

Other young women that I encountered had been targeted after an abuser saw them looking unhappy as they went to or came home from school, or saw that they were isolated and excluded from peer groups during break times.

Later, in practice, I encountered cases where young people felt confused by their sexuality and/or had experienced homophobia from friends, family and the community as a result of coming out. I also encountered young people who came from a different culture to the majority of young people in their community and felt that they were not welcome and did not fit in. There were also children from affluent families who were rebelling against parental control and plans for their future, along with academic pressures and expectations.

Common to all these cases is that all of the young people concerned were unhappy, isolated or seeking fulfilment or acknowledgement of their needs. This is what led me to question the relationship between perceived vulnerability and CSE, and the vulnerability that comes from day-to-day life – from just being a teenager, for example. We adults often forget how difficult and trying adolescence can be for the young person. The conclusion I arrived at was that some young people are in vulnerable situations and that this vulnerability can be identified and used to target and groom them. However, any young person can become vulnerable as a result of something that happens or has happened in their life; given a particular set of circumstances and opportunities, any young person can be vulnerable to becoming targeted and groomed. The key and necessary factor in all cases is opportunity. I will return to consider this later in the chapter.

Professional responses to child sexual exploitation

I then began to question the role of professionals and their responses to young people involved in CSE. Did their responses, assessments and interventions reduce or increase the vulnerability of the young people they were working with?

It is clear from national guidance and local Safeguarding Children Board policy throughout England and Wales that when CSE is identified as a risk factor for a young person, there should be a response from professionals involved that addresses and reduces risks. Best practice should involve looking at the 'push' and 'pull' factors, and reducing vulnerability and opportunities for them to be used as a means to target young people. Action should be taken to actively protect the young person; suspected abusers should be investigated and the abuse disrupted. Offering a therapeutic intervention reduces not only the young person's vulnerability but also the likelihood of their becoming a vulnerable adult. Preventative work is essential to raise the awareness of young people about risks that they may not know of and to which they would not know how to respond.

There have been some excellent practice responses to CSE. One example is Operation Retriever, a police operation launched in Derby in 2008.[7] Once victims had been identified and arrests made, a multi-agency team was established to run alongside the police investigation, with the young people and their welfare as the central focus. The young women received support from a specialist service, Safe and Sound, and also had access to therapeutic interventions. Their wider needs were identified and addressed. Relationships were established and built with the police. Any issues of witness intimidation were responded to promptly. The young women were supported and made to feel safe. Those who gave evidence at Crown Court, and ultimately saw their abusers convicted and imprisoned, did so with the support and active involvement of a range of professionals. The fact that a large number of young women felt able to give evidence against their abusers is evidence of how successful that intervention was. As is the fact that, some years later, a significant proportion of those young women were in education or employment. It is fair to say that these are young women who might in other circumstances have been regarded as 'damaged beyond repair' and certainly not able to lead 'normal' lives.

Normalising and validating abusive relationships

Over the years I have encountered outstanding practice like this, but more commonly I have experienced practice that I believe has increased young people's vulnerability and exposed them to greater risk and further harm. This has included normalising and validating relationships with abusers by, for example, referring to and regarding abusers as 'boyfriends' or 'sweethearts', or regarding relationships with older males as something 'that gay young men do'. I have seen abusers treated as if they were genuine partners of, or carers for, the children they were suspected of abusing.

Examples of this include abusers being invited to antenatal appointments, or being sent letters relating to a young person's education. In one case, a suspected abuser told the Risky Business project that he was contemplating seeking a residence order so that a young woman could officially live with him and he could claim child benefit for her. He claimed to be doing so with the support of local statutory services, and the project could find no information to contradict that. In another, more recent case, it was suggested to a parent that a child should remain with a suspected abuser because 'at least you know where she is – she isn't wandering the streets'. The reality in this case was that 'wandering the streets' might have been a far safer proposition for this young person.

Judging victims of CSE

I have encountered other examples of poor professional responses in the way that victims of CSE are regarded and judged. I have heard girls aged 12 referred to as 'promiscuous', 'a drama queen', 'a prostitute', 'attention seeking', 'streetwise', 'a fantasist', 'troubled', and the blame for their abuse laid firmly at their feet. Young people have been considered responsible for the abuse because they refused to make complaints to the police or to end the relationship with their abusers. Similarly, young people can be regarded as complicit in their own abuse because they return to abusers or continue to place themselves at risk. Failure to engage with professionals can be cited as a further reason to place responsibility for the abuse with the child.

When some of these cases so clearly crossed the thresholds for safeguarding responses or action by the police, I began to question the reasons for some of these responses and why those thresholds weren't being recognised in a significant number of cases. Sometimes it was because the young people didn't act like victims are supposed to. They were not 'nice' young people – often they were aggressive, verbally abusive, and involved in low-level criminality such as criminal damage or being drunk and disorderly. Sometimes they had been excluded from school because of their behaviour. Some were misusing alcohol and substances. In other words, helping them was a challenge; there was a perception that the help was not welcome and that scarce resources could be directed to other, more 'deserving' children. The act of non-engagement was seen as a legitimate reason for taking no further action. As one professional told me, 'If they won't help themselves, what are we expected to do about it?'

Understanding non-engagement

I want to explore some of the potential reasons for the non-engagement and some of these behaviours, because in most cases they were predictable and reasonable responses to unimaginable abuse. I believe that once you see CSE from the child's perspective, the question about non-engagement changes from 'Why won't they?' to 'Why would they?' There are several contributing factors to non-engagement and this is by no means an exhaustive consideration of all of those factors.

As already discussed in this chapter, child sexual exploitation is often a deeply sadistic form of abuse. It takes advantage of the vulnerability of young people, builds trust and hope, creates dependency, and then exposes the young person to multiple abuses, repeatedly and often over long periods of time. In this quote from her book, Emma Jackson describes the savagery of this type of abuse from the victim's perspective:

> Then he smiled his wide smile, which once I'd thought was charming and now looked plain evil. 'Don't forget your birthday present is waiting for you!' ... It was a few weeks before my fourteenth birthday ...
>
> 'I've got an idea for a present for you,' he announced. Despite everything, I still had a quick feeling of interest ... Still a kid I suppose. I couldn't resist asking, 'What?'
>
> He grinned. 'I'll line up every guy you've been with and let them do you, one another after another. You'll like that, won't you? Real birthday party. We can take photos.' And he laughed, but it wasn't an 'I'm-only-joking' laugh.[8]

Jenny Pearce and other researchers have talked about the identification of symptoms usually identified with post-traumatic stress syndrome in some of the young people who had been involved in CSE.[9] In cases of severe and sustained trauma, even the most balanced, intelligent and mature adult would struggle to function well, engage with services, and make the best decisions. If we reflect on our own personal histories most of us will have encountered trauma or stress, during which we may have made poor decisions, behaved less than perfectly, and struggled to function in our day-to-day lives. Why do we expect children, often damaged and vulnerable to begin with but certainly emotionally immature and now the victims of sustained abuse, to behave differently? How would most of us cope with the following scenarios?

J was taken to a bedroom and could hear a young woman screaming in apparent agony in the room next to her. She was told that the young person was being punished for not doing what her abusers wanted. The details of the punishment described to the young woman are too graphic to include here. The young woman was told that the same would happen to her if she failed to comply with what was being asked of her and if she told anyone anything about her abusers and what they were asking her to do.

T's young sister was enticed into a car with an abuser when T was trying to disengage from her abusers. T was told she had to make a choice, that she had to make it now and that the wrong choice would have severe and immediate consequences for her sister.

F's abuse was videoed and photographed and she was told it would be posted on the internet and shared with others such as family members and pupils at her school if she told anyone or failed to return the following evening.

Being involved in CSE unquestionably causes severe and significant trauma that impacts on every aspect of that young person's life – family, health, education, friendships, future prospects, mental health, and the relationships that they will have as an adult. This is considered repeatedly in research into CSE, and reflected in national policy and practice guidance. Involvement in CSE will cause deep-rooted trauma in most victims, which will be life-long and debilitating if not addressed. It is a vicious type of abuse and I often see the long-term effects when I am working with adults who were sexually exploited as children. I hesitate to call them 'survivors' as many of them are not surviving but fighting a daily battle just to face life. A good many have attempted suicide or expressed a desire to die. This account of the impact of her abuse given to me by one young woman demonstrates some of the reasons for this.

> It ruined my life. It stole my childhood from me. I can't get away from what he did to me. I can't trust anyone. I can't sleep. I can't love anyone or trust anyone. I'm afraid to go outside, not just because I might see him or some of the others, but how can I know who is safe? When I get on the bus, I think 'Did one of you rape me?' I never feel safe. Sometimes I want to go to sleep and never wake up, so I wouldn't have to deal with it anymore.

Engagement requires motivation and trust but in some cases the young people are unwilling or unable to give this. Engagement is sometimes scary and there is a risk that, if you share information about what has happened to you, there will be consequences. Information about you might be shared. You may lose control over what happens to you (i.e. where you live and who you live with). Your abuser may find out and you and/or others may be in danger. It also involves having to tell others about something that you want to forget ever happened. Often talking to one practitioner means being asked to tell others about the abuse.

There are also those young people who are in denial – that they have been groomed, that they are being abused, that the people they like and trust have betrayed them and always intended to do so. Some of the young people I work with have refused to believe that they are victims of abuse and that they are not in control of their situation. They have adopted distorted thinking – 'I want this,' 'I'm choosing to do this,' 'I'm getting something out of this,' 'I'm exploiting them' – to survive the best way that they can.

We also have to acknowledge that, for some young people, involvement in child sexual exploitation serves a purpose. It can make them feel real, alive, visible and relevant. The excitement of running away, of being where they shouldn't be, with people they shouldn't be with, is not to be underestimated – the pull of being with other young people and 'chilling', having access to alcohol and substances and sometimes being exposed to or involved in illegal activity. This can be exciting to young people at a developmental stage when they are given imperatives to take risks, to experiment and to reject authority and control. It is a stage where they are also seeking social acceptance and validation of their worth to others; a stage where they often want to feel part of something.

I have also observed that, when it comes to trauma, young people instinctively blame themselves. I have seen this in cases of domestic abuse, parental death, marriage breakdown, child abandonment, generic child abuse, and also in most cases involving CSE. Some of that in part seems to relate to what the young person was doing when they were first targeted – absent from school, for example, or involved in relationships or friendships that they knew their parents and carers were unlikely to approve of. Engaging in activities that they knew were wrong, such as drinking under age or using substances, can lead to guilt, and part of the grooming and control builds on and encourages this self-blame. Often professional responses can validate this belief and the young person's belief that no one will be able to prevent further abuse.

I have also seen professional responses to families become a factor in non-engagement. Concerned family members have become frustrated with the lack of response from statutory services when, for example, their child has gone missing from home. Even when they have been expressing concern about the people their children are with or houses they might be visiting that they believe are dangerous, they've been told that the police 'are not a taxi service' or told to go and look for their child themselves. Children who go missing repeatedly have sometimes been regarded as less of a concern because their family has known where they are or who they are with. In a number of cases in which I have been involved, a potential abuser has been deemed a protective factor, which is extremely worrying. Families have been reminded of their parental responsibility and how they have a duty to keep their children safe. In some of those cases it was the parents who initiated professional involvement with their families because they could not keep their children safe and were asking for help in doing so. Where families raised objections to professional responses (often in less-than-diplomatic terms due to worry, fear and frustration) they too were labelled – as 'troubled' families, as somehow less deserving of help and support than other, less aggressive parents. This, combined with the behaviour of the child, often resulted in them being labelled 'hard to engage' or 'resistant to working with services'. I often read case files and wondered if, as a parent in the same situation, my response would be any different.

My experience of professional responses has been that often young people involved in CSE are judged on their actions and their behaviours – without anyone questioning the cause or trying to see it from the child's perspective to understand the 'why'. Responses to trauma often manifest as asocial behaviour. Responding to the behaviour without understanding its causes has the consequence that any professional assessment fails to recognise the young person as a victim of abuse and/ or in need of help or resources. The result has been that victims of abuse are left to make decisions about their lives that ultimately place them at risk of further abuse. An example is the case of L.

L was 14 when was she was groomed by K, an adult male. Initially her mother regarded K as a positive influence on her daughter; she later became concerned about the amount of time L was spending with him and began to question the relationship. L admitted to her mother that she was having a sexual relationship with K. She told her mother that she would be leaving home at 16 and going to live with K. L's mother involved social care and the police but, as L was approaching 16, her mother was told that the relationship was clearly consensual and there was nothing anyone could do about it as her daughter was unwilling to make a complaint that she had been abused. K was significantly older than L, and concerns about his relationships with young vulnerable girls had been expressed in the past.

It can be seen how the issue of the young person's apparent consent (even though she was below the legal age of consent) clouded the real issues of this case. This was a significantly older male who had a previous allegation of sexual abuse made against him – a man who had acted in a predatory way, gaining a vulnerable young woman's confidence and trust, building on her interests and encouraging a sexual relationship that no reasonable adult would think acceptable. The professional response reinforced K's power and control over L, and also removed protective factors. It left L's mother powerless to protect her. L's mother filed an official complaint but by the time it was considered L was over 16. L's mother was told that there was no further action that could be taken, unless her daughter made a complaint. This was despite L still being considered a child under the Children Act 1989, and that the definition of child sexual exploitation includes children up to their eighteenth birthday. There was evidence that L had been targeted, groomed and involved in sexual activity while under 16 years of age. Nevertheless L's case was closed.

I believe the professional response in L's case essentially allowed her to make unchallenged decisions about her life that resulted in her continuing abuse. L's mother currently has no contact with her daughter.

Created vulnerability and opportunities to abuse

Professional responses such as these increase a young person's vulnerability as often the power of the abuser is strengthened and reinforced. Some young people believe that there is no alternative. Consider the following young people and how the professional responses in each case increased their vulnerability.

> Q was visited by the police at her 'boyfriend's' flat after concerns about possible abuse had been reported to the police. She was asked if she was safe and well – in the presence of the adult suspected of abusing her. Her affirmative answer was accepted without challenge because Q had been given an opportunity to tell the professional concerned if she was worried or if anyone was abusing her (even though this was in the presence of her abuser).

P's mother, grandmother and younger sister were threatened with rape when P started attending a specialist project. P told a practitioner about this, who sought advice from social care and the police. She was told not to worry; it was 'probably just empty threats'.

N's sibling was subjected to a severe physical attack by multiple perpetrators and needed inpatient hospital treatment as a result of injuries he sustained.

M's house was subject to criminal damage. The family was offered a panic button and extra door locks. The person who the family thought was responsible for this and for abusing their daughter was not questioned by police.

When Z made a complaint to the police, her family were told that it was her word against her abusers and that she would have a traumatic time at court. She was later told that the police were considering charging her with wasting police time.

G made a complaint to the police and agreed to be medically examined. On the way to the hospital a professional talked her out of proceeding with the complaint, telling her that G was 'not very believable' and 'really it is just your word against his'. G's complaint was against a man about whom repeated concerns and information suggesting an involvement in CSE had been shared with the police.

Some young people talked about the likely costs of not obeying their abusers or of engaging with professionals. As one young woman said to her foster carer who was trying to prevent her leaving the home, 'You don't know what will happen to me if I don't go.' Another young woman said, 'The consequences of not complying, what they would do, was so much worse than what they were going to do anyway that I learned the best way to protect myself was to do as I was told.'

Professional perceptions of child sexual exploitation as a child protection issue

One of the difficulties has been how child sexual exploitation has been and continues to be perceived by some professionals. The term used to be 'child prostitution' – and this is still used in current legislation, such as the Sexual Offences Act 2003. Awareness of CSE is still in the early stages among many practitioners and services. It is a complex, challenging, upsetting and abhorrent type of abuse and young people involved in it are unlikely to engage with services, as discussed previously. It is resource intensive and there are no 'quick fixes'. I think we have to acknowledge that a combination of these factors, along with increasing workloads, lack of awareness, and lack of recognition that this is a child protection issue all contribute to the inadequacy of professional responses.

What is certain, however, is that by failing to understand the reasons for young people's behaviour and the decisions they are apparently making of their own free will, and by failing to find out the reasons for that behaviour and those decisions, professional responses can increase their vulnerability. The consequence is that young people are made more accessible to abusers, the power and control process is easier for abusers to apply and, while young people and their carers are less able to protect themselves, they are subject to continuing and often increasingly violent abuse that damages them for life.

Towards best practice

In this chapter I have considered how vulnerability is something that any young person can experience. While it is a factor in young people becoming involved in CSE, another key issue is opportunity. The response of professionals can decrease risk factors and opportunities but it can also increase them by normalising and validating abusive relationships, focusing on young people's behaviours and choices, and failing to see child sexual exploitation as child abuse and a child protection issue.

The challenge for future practice is recognising these shortcomings and addressing them. Best practice:

- recognises and responds to the abuse as a child protection issue
- focuses on the behaviour of the abusers, not the victims
- recognises and understands issues of vulnerability, and considers how to deliver preventative work that addresses and reduces risk
- understands the impact of trauma on behaviour
- acknowledges the relationship between professional responses and future vulnerability
- identifies failure to engage as an additional risk factor

- ensures that legal processes, especially those involving giving evidence at court, are more supportive and victim focused.

Until we have these practices embedded in our responses to CSE, vulnerability will remain unaddressed and, exacerbated by poor professional responses, continue to result in young people being identified, targeted, groomed and sexually, emotionally and physically abused.

Endnotes

1. Vulnerability can be seen as a situational rather than dispositional state. For further discussion of the concept of vulnerability see Chapters 1 and 2 in this volume.
2. Department for Education (2009). *Safeguarding Children and Young People from Sexual Exploitation.* London: Department for Education. https://www.gov.uk/government/publications/safeguarding-children-and-young-people-from-sexual-exploitation-supplementary-guidance (retrieved 10 September, 2015).
3. See Jay, A. (2014). *Independent Inquiry into Child Sexual Exploitation in Rotherham (1997–2013).* Rotherham: Rotherham Metropolitan Borough Council. www.rotherham.gov.uk/downloads/file/1407/independent_inquiry_cse_in_rotherham (retrieved 9 September, 2015).
4. Casey, L. (2015). *Inspection into the Governance of Rotherham Council.* London: Department for Communities and Local Government. www.gov.uk/government/collections/inspection-into-the-governance-of-rotherham-council (retrieved 9 September, 2015).
5. All the examples given in this chapter are composites taken from a larger sample of children and young people. A colleague involved in the project has reviewed the examples for identifiability and confirmed the anonymity of the children and families.
6. Gillick competence is a term originating in England and is used in medical law to decide whether a child (aged 16 years or younger) is deemed able to consent to his or her own medical treatment without the need for parental permission or knowledge.
7. See Derby City Council (undated). *Child Sexual Exploitation.* [Online] www.derby.gov.uk/health-and-social-care/safeguarding-children/child-sexual-exploitation/ (retrieved 9 September, 2015).
8. Jackson, E. (2010). *The End of My World.* London: Ebury Press, p.229.
9. See, for example, Melrose, M., Pearce, J. (eds) (2013). *Critical Perspectives on Child Sexual Exploitation and Related Trafficking.* Basingstoke: Palgrave Macmillan.

Part two
Just services?

Chapter 7
The rights of parents and children in regard to children receiving psychiatric diagnoses and drugs

Peter R. Breggin

This chapter asks whether it is ever in the best interests of a child to be given a psychiatric diagnosis or drug. It also asks whether a parent under any circumstance should be forced to accept a psychiatric diagnosis or a drug for a child. For practical purposes the focus is on the diagnosis attention deficit hyperactivity disorder (ADHD) and stimulant drugs, and on the diagnosis bipolar disorder and antipsychotic (neuroleptic) drugs. The conclusion is that there are always better alternatives to the psychiatric diagnosis and medication of children, and that society should find a way to ban these approaches in regard to children.

Setting standards for the protection of children
Although the US Senate has refused to ratify the UN Convention on the Rights of the Child, many federal and state laws and legal precedents have established a broad array of commonly enforced protections and rights for children in the US.[1] Some rights are common for every child. These include the right to a safe environment, good nutrition, healthcare and education. A child's need for safety even trumps the parents' rights to care for their child, and allows the state to take children away from their parents if the parents are not meeting their basic needs.[2] Children also have selected constitutional rights, including some of the protections enumerated in the Bill of Rights. Specifically, they have the right to equal protection, which means that every child is entitled to the same treatment at the hands of authority regardless of race, gender, disability or religion. Laws relating to special education are an effort to accommodate children with disabilities and ensure that they receive

the same education as their peers. Children are entitled to due process, which includes notice and a hearing, before any of their basic rights are taken away by the government.[3]

US courts rely upon the standard of the child's best interests.[4] These standards include the 'the physical, mental, emotional and moral wellbeing' of the child, a standard I shall use in this analysis.[5]

Children's rights in regard to medical treatment

Every US state makes provision for the termination of parental rights if they fail to take care of their child's best interests. Grounds for termination include severe or chronic abuse or neglect, abandonment, parental disabilities that interfere with raising the children, and the failure to provide adequate medical care.

Concern for the best interests of children has led to interventions by child protective services and family courts to force parents to provide unwanted medical care to their children. For example, parents have been forced to provide generally accepted medical treatment for childhood leukemia.[6] I have been a medical expert on behalf of parents whose children have been forced to take psychiatric medications as a result of court interventions brought against them by the other parent, child protective health services and state mental health authorities.[7]

In regard to psychiatric treatment, what is the child's best interest?

This chapter will examine two questions from the viewpoint of the child's best interests. First, 'Is it in any child's best interest to have a psychiatric diagnosis, such as ADHD, oppositional defiant disorder (ODD), autism, bipolar disorder or even a learning disorder (LD) such as dyslexia?' Second, 'Is it in any child's best interest to be treated with a psychiatric drug, such as a stimulant, benzodiazepine, antidepressant, mood stabiliser or antipsychotic drug?' In addition, this analysis will address the question, 'Should a parent under any circumstances be forced to accept a psychiatric diagnosis for a child and/or the administration of a psychiatric drug to a child, even if medical specialists believe the child needs the diagnosis or treatment?'

For practical purposes, the focus will be on stimulant and antipsychotic drugs, but all psychiatric drugs are hazardous for children. For example, routine treatment with antidepressants can cause severe behavioural abnormalities, violence and even suicide in children.[8]

Effects of the ADHD diagnosis and stimulant drugs

The myth of ADHD

ADHD is not a valid diagnostic category that meets the criteria for a medical syndrome.[9] Like all other psychiatric disorders, there is no evidence that it is caused by a biochemical imbalance.[10] The three ADHD behavioural categories of hyperactivity, impulsivity and inattention do not reflect an underlying syndrome or known biological or genetic cause. Sometimes these behaviours are part of normal childhood development. At other times they result from boring and poorly disciplined classrooms, lack of grade-level educational skills, emotional difficulties generated from problems at home or in school, hunger or poor nutrition, insomnia and fatigue, and a variety of chronic illnesses, including diabetes and head injury (e.g. sports concussions). In my clinical practice, the causes are usually an educational misfit or inadequate discipline at home, or both. Among children in poverty, common environmental causes range from head injury and malnutrition to chaotic family life.[11]

The class of stimulant drugs

Stimulants are the most commonly prescribed drugs for ADHD. Most are either amphetamines (e.g. Adderall or Dexedrine) or methylphenidate (e.g. Ritalin or Concerta). Based on their pharmacological similarity, the labels for drugs containing methylphenidate should be nearly identical to those for amphetamines, but the methylphenidate labels are weaker in regard to their warnings due to inadequacies in the US Food and Drug Administration (FDA) updating of old labels.[12]

Atomoxetine (Strattera) has been promoted by manufacturer Eli Lilly and Co. as a 'non-stimulant' treatment for ADHD. It is not a classic stimulant because it lacks typical abuse potential. It does, however, cause dangerously stimulating symptoms in one-third of children.[13] Strattera carries a 'black box' warning about causing suicidality in children.[14]

Dependence (addiction) and abuse

Amphetamine and methylphenidate belong to the Drug Enforcement Agency's (DEA) Schedule II, which is the highest level of risk of addiction and abuse. The black box warning at the top of the Adderall label should also apply to the methylphenidate products.[15]

> WARNING: POTENTIAL FOR ABUSE
>
> Amphetamines have a high potential for abuse. Administration of amphetamines for prolonged periods of time may lead to drug dependence. Pay particular attention to the possibility of subjects obtaining amphetamines for non-therapeutic use or distribution to others and these drugs should be prescribed or dispensed sparingly [see DRUG ABUSE AND DEPENDENCE (9)].
>
> Misuse of amphetamines may cause sudden death and serious cardiovascular adverse reactions.

Predisposing to drug abuse in young adulthood

Lambert conducted a 28-year prospective study of children diagnosed with ADHD. She found that children treated with methylphenidate were much more likely to abuse cocaine in young adulthood compared with those diagnosed with ADHD without drug exposure.[16] This is not surprising, since stimulants cause physical alterations in the reward centres of the brain.[17]

Methylphenidate, amphetamine, methamphetamine and cocaine are so similar pharmacologically that animals and humans will cross-addict to all of them.[18]

Brain damage and dysfunction

Amphetamine and methylphenidate produce persistent and sometimes permanent biochemical abnormalities in the brain.[19] Children treated with stimulants often develop atrophy of the brain. At the NIH Consensus Development Conference on ADHD, Swanson and Castellanos reviewed available studies purporting to show biological bases for ADHD including brain atrophy.[20,21] My presentation at the same conference concluded that these brain scans were 'almost certainly measuring pathology caused by psychostimulants'.[22] Similarly, Proal and colleagues found widespread brain atrophy in adults who had been diagnosed and treated for ADHD as children.[23]

Growth suppression

A large-scale federally-funded study involving multiple centres, the Multimodal Treatment Study (MTA), reconfirmed that stimulants suppress growth.[24] These stimulant-induced losses in growth are due to a disruption in growth hormone cycles that could adversely affect other organs of the body.[25]

Depression and apathy induced by stimulants

A study of children aged four to six given methylphenidate found that two-thirds developed symptoms of depression and withdrawal.[26] Older children could also become 'tired, withdrawn, listless, depressed, dopey, dazed, subdued and inactive'.[27] When these adverse drug effects are mistaken for a worsening of the child's 'mental disorders', these children are often given more serious diagnoses and additional drugs, leading to chronicity.

Obsessive-compulsive conduct and tics induced by stimulants

An NIMH study focused on stimulant-induced symptoms of obsessive compulsive disorder (OCD) and found that 51 per cent of methylphenidate-treated children were afflicted with drug-induced OCD.[28] The study also found that 58 per cent of methylphenidate-treated children developed abnormal movements, usually tics. The authors believed that the OCD symptoms and the tics were functionally related in drug-induced brain dysfunction.

How stimulants work

Numerous animal studies confirm that stimulant drugs produce apathy or indifference, plus obsessive-like meaningless behaviours.[29] Consistent with the brain-disabling principle of psychiatric drug effects, this production of depression and apathy is the primary or 'therapeutic' effect.[30] The drug-induced reduction in spontaneous behaviour and enforcement of obsessive behaviour appears beneficial to teachers and parents who are struggling to handle difficult, active, bored or upset children. The more listless and compulsive child requires much less attention in school or at home. Motivation to socialise or to otherwise get into trouble is diminished.

Discouraging the development of self-control and self-determination

When children are told they have ADHD they are given the idea that they cannot control their behaviour. This undermines their sense of responsibility and self-determination. Normal child development requires, perhaps above all else, that children learn to take increasing responsibility for their conduct. The diagnosis of ADHD discourages personal responsibility, and the stimulant drugs crush the ability to exercise it.

Effectiveness

No long-term benefit for children of any kind has ever been demonstrated for any stimulant drug – no improved behaviour, no improved socialisation skills, no improved academic skills and no improvement in learning. There is no longer any need to repeat my lengthy analysis in *Brain-Disabling Treatments in Psychiatry*.[31] The extremely pro-medication Multi-Modal Treatment Study (MTA) came to these same negative conclusions as earlier studies. At 36 months, medication treatment strategies were no better than any other behavioural and educational approaches, including a brief stay at a summer camp.[32] But the children were smaller in stature.[33]

'Antipsychotic' drugs

The antipsychotic drugs include older ones such as chlorpromazine (Thorazine), haloperidol (Haldol) and perphenazine (Trilafon), as well as the newer 'atypicals' or 'novel' antipsychotic drugs such as olanzapine (Zyprexa), risperidone (Risperdal), aripiprazole (Abilify), ziprasidone (Geodon) and quetiapine (Seroquel). There are four yet newer atypical antipsychotics: paliperidone (Invega), iloperidone (Fanapt), lurasidone (Latuda) and asenapine (Saphris).

All of these drugs disrupt dopamine neurotransmission (that is, they are D_2 blockers).[34] Therefore they will cause the same adverse effects as the older antipsychotic drugs, including lobotomy-like indifference and apathy, Parkinsonian symptoms, akathisia, dystonia, tardive dyskinesia, neuroleptic malignant syndrome, gynecomastia, and other sexual dysfunctions. The atypicals also impact on numerous other neurotransmitter systems, including serotonin, and all can cause a metabolic syndrome (see below).

Tardive dyskinesia, tardive dystonia and tardive akathisia

Tardive dyskinesia (TD) is a movement disorder caused by antipsychotic drugs (dopamine blockers). It can impair any muscle functions that are wholly or partially under voluntary control, including the face, eyes, tongue, jaw, neck, back abdomen, extremities, diaphragm, oesophagus, and vocal cords. Dozens of controlled clinical trials and epidemiological studies demonstrate that the rates for tardive dyskinesia are an astronomical five to eight per cent cumulative per year.[35]

Tardive akathisia, a variant of TD, causes a torture-like inner agitation that typically compels its sufferers into physical motion. This disorder frequently drives patients into despair, and even into psychosis.[36] Tardive dystonia, another variant, causes painful and deforming spasms.

All antipsychotic drugs can cause every variation of TD and all carry the same or similar TD warning on their FDA-approved labels. If study subjects are given equivalent doses of the older and newer antipsychotic drugs, there is little or no difference in the frequency of extrapyramidal effects or TD.[37] The NIMH-sponsored Clinical Antipsychotic Trials of Intervention Effectiveness (CATIE) study found that 'There were no statistically significant differences between the rates of extrapyramidal side effects, movement disorders, or akathisia.'[38] A study in 2010 looked at 352 patients who were initially free of TD, finding little difference in TD rates between the atypical and classic neuroleptics, with an average range of approximately five per cent per year.[39]

Neuroleptic malignant syndrome (NMS) closely resembles viral encephalitis, leaving many survivors with cognitive deficits and TD. Again caused by so-called antipsychotic drugs (actually major tranquillisers), NMS appears in recipients at a rate of one to two per cent or more per year and can be fatal in 20 per cent of untreated cases.[40]

Children and TD

Psychiatric Drugs: Hazards to the brain features the first detailed review demonstrating that tardive dyskinesia is a major threat to children.[41] The issue is no longer in doubt. In my clinical and forensic practice, I have evaluated dozens of cases of childhood TD caused by 'atypicals' including risperidone, olanzapine, ziprasidone, aripiprazole and quetiapine.

Shrinkage of the brain (atrophy)

Evidence for antipsychotic drugs causing brain damage began to accumulate decades ago.[42]

Recent brain scan studies confirm that exposure to antipsychotic drugs causes brain shrinkage (atrophy) in patients.[43] Shrinkage of brain tissue has also been demonstrated in primates.[44] Many studies show underlying cellular damage in the brain and body.[45]

Tardive psychosis and tardive dementia

Referring to studies of tardive dyskinesia in both children and adults, Gualtieri and Barnhill concluded, 'In virtually every clinical survey that has addressed the question, it is found that TD patients, compared to non-TD patients, have more in the way of dementia.'[46] Patients withdrawn from antipsychotic drugs have often been made more disturbed and psychotic (tardive psychosis) than before they took the medications.[47] Children manifest tardive psychosis as a severe worsening of their behaviour beyond pretreatment intensity.[48] Long-term patients can develop neuroleptic-induced deficit syndrome (NIDS) with cognitive and affective losses leading to a diagnosis of chronic schizophrenia.[49]

Metabolic syndrome

The newer antipsychotics cause a metabolic syndrome that predisposes to heart disease and early death. The syndrome includes weight gain and obesity, elevated blood sugar and diabetes, elevated blood lipids and atherosclerosis, and high blood pressure. Along with the additional risk of pancreatitis and cardiac arrhythmia, antipsychotic drugs produce potentially fatal risks and shorten lifespan. The CATIE study found that the prevalence of metabolic syndrome was over 40 per cent, including more than 50 per cent of the females.[50] One-third or more of children and adolescents given antipsychotic drugs are at risk of developing metabolic syndrome.[51]

Bipolar disorder and the increasing prescription of antipsychotic drugs to children

Moreno and colleagues reported a 40-fold increase in the diagnosis of childhood bipolar disorder between 1994–1995 and 2002–2003. A remarkable 90.6 per cent of the children received psychiatric drugs, and 47.7 per cent were prescribed antipsychotic drugs.[52] Joseph Biederman, Thomas Spencer and Timothy Wilens from Harvard fuelled this increase in diagnosing and drugging children while accepting funds from the pharmaceutical industry in return for promoting their products.[53] The problem of over-medicating children has drawn some attention.[54] After deliberation, the authors of the American Psychiatric Association's *Diagnostic and Statistical Manual of Mental Disorders, Fifth Edition: DSM-5* decided not to include childhood bipolar disorder among official diagnoses, but this will probably do little to slow down the epidemic drugging of children with antipsychotic drugs.

Increased mortality and shortened lifespan

Patients diagnosed with mental disorders have a markedly shortened lifespan: as much as 13.8 years among US Veterans Administration patients and 25 years in state mental health systems.[55] Most of these patients have had years of antipsychotic drug exposure. Adults aged 20 to 34 on antidepressants have increased mortality when also taking antipsychotic drugs or mood stabilisers, excluding lithium.[56] The increased mortality is not related to lifestyle but to polydrug treatment.[57]

Efficacy of 'antipsychotic' medications

Antipsychotic drugs have their 'therapeutic' effect by suppressing the frontal lobes and reticular activating system, producing relative degrees of apathy and docility.[58] The drugs have the same impact on people regardless of diagnosis and, indeed, the same impact on animals.[59]

The CATIE study gives a bleak picture of antipsychotic drug efficacy. It found: 'In summary, patients with chronic schizophrenia in this study discontinued their antipsychotic study medications at a high rate, indicating substantial limitations in the effectiveness of the drugs.'[60] The two lead authors of the CATIE study, Lieberman and Stroup, concluded, 'By revealing the truth about the emperor's new clothes, CATIE has helped to refocus efforts on the need for truly innovative treatments and strategies that can make significant advances for persons with schizophrenia and related psychoses.'[61] The two authors note that 'prescribing patterns have not markedly changed' despite the results of the CATIE study.[62] The CATIE results are consistent with decades of research confirming the lack of efficacy of antipsychotic drugs.[63]

These same concerns should be expressed about the administration of *any* psychiatric drug to children, as exemplified by the supposedly less dangerous stimulants which were evaluated in the previous section.[64]

The harm of diagnosing and psychiatrically drugging children

Children are stigmatised, potentially for life, with diagnoses that have considerable prejudice attached to them in society, causing loss of self-esteem and bringing disadvantages in regard to their future opportunities. They are influenced to view themselves falsely as physically or genetically disabled, leading to feelings of dependency and helplessness, and a lack of self-determination or personal responsibility. At the same time, the diagnoses encourage reliance on psychiatric medication, too often leading to lifetime exposure to toxic chemicals.

No psychiatric drugs have been proven effective for children, long-term (i.e. for many months or years). Prescribing these drugs to children not only exposes them to very serious adverse effects and shortened lives; it also diverts attention from the child's real needs and from better, psychosocial and educational approaches.

The use of psychiatric drugs, similar to psychiatric labelling, exposes the child to stigmatisation. It leads to loss of self-esteem, causes feelings of dependency and helplessness, and enforces psychological dependency on psychiatry and on psychoactive substances. The drugged child's brain cannot develop normally and instead will develop in response to a toxic internal environment. This robs the child of the opportunity to grow up as determined by his or her genetic endowment. The child instead grows up physically and mentally affected by the medication in ways that can never be fully understood, and without achieving his or her maximum potential.

Finally, when children are exposed to psychiatric drugs for several years, injuries to brain function can make it impossible for the now young adult to stop taking them.

Psychiatric drugs do much more harm than good in treating children. Nor will improvements in psychopharmacology significantly improve the risk/benefit ratio. The problems that children face are psychological, social, educational and moral in nature. Psychiatric diagnoses cannot possibly capture the richness and complexity, the human quality, of what the child is experiencing. Psychiatric drugs cannot touch the underlying problems; they can only temporarily suppress their manifestations, while adding brain impairments.

Answers to the specific questions

The first question was: 'Is it in any child's best interest to have a psychiatric diagnosis, such as ADHD, oppositional defiant disorder (ODD), autism, bipolar disorder or even a learning disorder (LD) such as dyslexia?' The answer to this question is 'no'. Psychiatric diagnoses lack a scientific basis and pigeonhole children. Instead, every effort must be directed to understanding and meeting the psychosocial and educational needs of each individual child.

The second question was: 'Is it in any child's best interest to be treated with a psychiatric drug, such as a stimulant, benzodiazepine, antidepressant, mood stabiliser or antipsychotic drug?' The answer is 'no'. Psychiatric drugs cause considerable harm to the brain and mind of the child, and cannot directly address any of the child's actual problems.

The additional question was: 'Should a parent under any circumstances be forced to accept a psychiatric diagnosis for a child or the administration of a psychiatric drug to a child, even if medical specialists believe the child needs the diagnosis or treatment?' The answer to this is 'no'. Because of the inevitability of drug-induced harm to the child's brain, parents should never be forced to accept a psychiatric diagnosis or medication for their child.

Medical versus psychiatric medications

There are circumstances when psychoactive substances have a legitimate medical purpose in the treatment of children, such as surgical anaesthesia, relief of physical pain and control of seizures. These *medical* drugs (in contrast to *psychiatric* drugs) are not intended for the control of behaviour and emotions, or the treatment of psychiatric disorders. (Nonetheless, even in these cases, great caution should be used if and when children are exposed to chemicals that affect the brain.)

This distinction between medical drugs and psychiatric drugs is similar to one that I first made in the early 1970s when delineating the difference between genuine *neurosurgery*, for the treatment of physical disorders such as seizures, and *psychosurgery* or *psychiatric surgery* for the control of emotions and behaviour and the treatment of psychiatric disorders. These distinctions between genuine neurosurgery and psychosurgery were used in legislation in the early 1970s by the US Congress, including the creation of the Psychosurgery Commission.[65] They were also used in the judicial opinion in Kaimowitz v. Department of Mental Health, a landmark psychosurgery case in which I offered these distinctions during my testimony.[66] The Kaimowitz decision contributed to ending psychosurgery in US state hospitals, the Veterans Administration, and the National Institutes of Health (NIH). It is time to apply these distinctions in regard to the epidemic of psychiatric drugging of children throughout the Western world to curtail and eventually end the use of psychoactive substances to control emotions and behaviour in children.

The child's right to be free of psychoactive substances

All children exposed to psychiatric diagnoses and drugs will suffer impairment of their 'physical, mental, emotional and moral wellbeing' (see introduction to this chapter). Impairment of *physical* wellbeing is inevitable. All psychiatric drugs impair brain function. They also impair overall physical health, leading to, for example, stunting of growth (stimulants) and metabolic syndrome (antipsychotic drugs).

Impairment of *mental* and *emotional* functions inevitably follows from the brain-disabling effects of the drug. For example, the stimulants and the so-called antipsychotic drugs work by producing diminished spontaneity and social interest, often leading to apathy or depression.

Impairment of *moral* functioning is inevitable. Stimulants, antipsychotic drugs, and all other psychiatric drugs impair frontal lobe function, compromising empathy and social relationships.[67] In addition, psychiatric drugs impair judgement, impulse control and other aspects of moral capacity.

Prolonged exposure to psychiatric drugs frequently leads to brain shrinkage and chronic brain impairment (CBI) with cognitive dysfunction, apathy, emotional instability and impaired judgement.[68] This, too, threatens the child's 'physical, mental, emotional and moral wellbeing'.

Even if some evidence could be generated in the future for the effectiveness of psychiatric drugs in the treatment of children, the much more obvious, demonstrable and dominant adverse effects would necessitate protecting children from them.

Because they do not address the child's real issues or problems, and because they inevitably harm the child, the following conclusions can be drawn:

Psychoactive drugs should not be given to children for the purpose of controlling their emotions or behaviour, or for treating psychiatric diagnoses or disorders. It is the right of every child to be protected from psychoactive chemicals administered for psychiatric purposes.

Implementing every child's right to be free of psychiatric drugs is, of course, a huge and complex, long-term undertaking. Stopping short of a ban, attorney Jim Gottstein has described some of the possible legal steps in protecting children.[69] Any significant reduction in the widespread drugging of children will cut deeply into the authority, power and profits of the entire psychopharmaceutical complex from drug companies and medical societies to individual researchers and prescribers, and will therefore meet enormous resistance.[70] Protecting children from psychiatric medications will require a transformation of society based on addressing their genuine needs. We begin this transformation by declaring the principle that every child has the right to grow up with a brain free of psychoactive substances, including psychiatric drugs.

As a start, individual parents should avoid putting their children on psychiatric drugs and, if already on drugs, parents should seek help in withdrawing them as soon and as safely as possible.[71] Physicians and other prescribers should resist every pressure to put children on psychiatric medications and instead work towards withdrawing them from these drugs as soon and as safely as possible.

Hopefully society will learn to view the psychiatric diagnosing and drugging of children as a huge and tragic mistake. Hopefully society will realise that the interests of children are best served by ending the use of psychiatric diagnoses and psychiatric medications, while turning attention towards psychosocial, family and educational approaches that meet the genuine needs of children.

Acknowledgement

This is an expanded version of a paper first appearing in *Children and Society*, May, 2014. Sections are reprinted with the kind permission of John Wiley & Sons.

Endnotes

1. UNICEF (n.d.). Convention on the Rights of the Child. Available at http://www.unicef.org/crc (retrieved 19 January 2013); Gottstein, J. (2012). Legal issues surrounding the psychiatric drugging of children and youth. In: S. Olfman & B. Robbins (Eds). *Drugging our Children: How profiteers are pushing antipsychotics on our youngest and what we can do to stop it* (pp. 99–115). Santa Barbara, CA: Praeger.
2. FindLaw (n.d.). What are the legal rights of children? Available at http://family.findlaw.com/emancipation-of-minors/what-are-the-legal-rights-of-children.html (retrieved 19 January 2013).
3. Ibid.
4. Child Welfare Information Gateway (2012). Determining the best interests of the child: Summary of state laws. Washington, DC: Administration for Children & Families and US Department of Health & Human Services. Available at https://www.childwelfare.gov/topics/systemwide/laws-policies/statutes/best-interest/?hasBeenRedirected=1 (retrieved 19 January 2013).
5. FindLaw, What are the legal rights of children? See note 2 ; FindLaw (n.d.). Terminating parental rights. Available at http://family.findlaw.com/parental-rights-and-liability/terminating-parental-rights.html (retrieved 20 January 2013); Child Welfare Information Gateway, 201. See note 4. See also Gottstein, 2012. See note 1.
6. CBS News (2012). Minn. court intervenes when family refuses daughter's chemo. Available at http://www.cbsnews.com/8301-201_162-57488583/minn-court-intervenes-when-family-refuses-daughters-chemo/ (retrieved 19 January 2013); Gottstein, 2012. See note 1.
7. Breggin, P. (2008a). *Medication Madness: The role of psychiatric drugs in cases of violence, suicide, and crime*. New York: St. Martin's Press.
8. Breggin, P. (2008b). *Brain-disabling Treatments in Psychiatry: Drugs, electroshock, and the psychopharmaceutical complex* (2nd edition). New York: Springer Publishing Company; Breggin, 2008a. See note 7; Breggin, P. (2010). Antidepressant-induced suicide, violence, and mania: Risks for military personnel. *Ethical Human Psychology and Psychiatry*, 12, 111–121.
9. Baughman, F. & Hovey, C. (2006). *The ADHD Fraud: How psychiatry makes 'patients' of normal children*. Victoria, BC, Canada: Trafford Publishing; Breggin, 2008b. See note 8.
10. Moncrieff, J. (2008). *The Myth of the Chemical Cure: A critique of psychiatric drug treatment*. Basingstoke: Palgrave Macmillan.
11. Breggin, P. & Breggin, G. (1998). *The War Against Children of Color: Psychiatry targets inner city children*. Monroe, ME: Common Courage Press.

12. Breggin, 2008b. See note 8.
13. Henderson, T. A. & Hartman, K. (2004). Aggression, mania, and hypomania induction associated with atomoxetine. *Pediatrics, 114*, 895–896.
14. PDR Network (2011). Strattera. In *Physicians' Desk Reference*. Montvale, NJ: PDR Network.
15. Shire (2011). Adderall: Complete prescribing information and medication guide. Available at http://www.shire.com/shireplc/en/investors/irshirenews?id=544 (retrieved 20 January 2013).
16. Lambert, N. (2005). The contribution of childhood ADHD, conduct problems, and stimulant treatment to adolescent and adult tobacco and psychoactive substance abuse. *Ethical Human Psychology and Psychiatry, 7*, 197–221.
17. Carlezon, W. & Konradi, C. (2004). Understanding the neurobiological consequences of early exposure to psychotropic drugs: Linking behaviour with molecules. *Neuropharmacology, 47* (Suppl. 1) 46–60.
18. Breggin, 2008b. See note 8.
19. Ibid., pp. 307–317.
20. Swanson, J. & Castellanos, F. (1998). Biological bases of attention deficit hyperactivity disorder: Neuroanatomy, genetics, and pathophysiology. In: *NIH Consensus Development Conference Program and Abstracts: Diagnosis and treatment of attention deficit hyperactivity disorder* (pp. 37–42). Rockville, MD: National Institutes of Health.
21. Castellanos, F. X., Giedd, J., Marsh, W., Hamburger, S., Vaituzis, A., Dickstein, D., et al. (1998). Quantitative brain magnetic resonance imaging in attention-deficit hyperactivity disorder. *Archives of General Psychiatry, 53*, 607–616; Giedd, J. N., Castellanos, F. X., Casey, B. J., Kozuch, P., King, A. C., Hamburger, S. D. & Rapoport, J. (1994). Quantitative morphology of the corpus callosum in attention deficit hyperactivity disorder. *American Journal of Psychiatry, 151*, 665–669.
22. Breggin, P. (1998). Risks and mechanism of action of stimulants. In *NIH Consensus Development Conference program and abstracts: Diagnosis and treatment of attention deficit hyperactivity disorder* (pp. 105–120). Rockville, MD: National Institutes of Health, p. 109.
23. Proal, E., Reiss, P., Klein, R., Mannuzza, S., Gotimer, K., Ramos-Olazagasti, M., Lerch, J., He, Y., Zijdenbos, A., Kelly, C., Milham, M. & Castellanos, F. X. (2011). Brain gray matter deficits at 33-year follow-up in adults with attention-deficit/hyperactivity disorder established in childhood. *Archives of General Psychiatry, 68*, 1122–1134.
24. Swanson, J., Elliott. G., Greenhill, L., Wigal, T., Arnold, L., Vitiello, B., Hechtman, L., Epstein, J., Pelham, W., Abikoff, H., Newcorn, J., Molina, B., Hinshaw, S., Wells, K., Hoza, B., Jensen, P., Gibbons, R., Hur, K., Stehli, A., Davies, M., March, J., Conners, C., Caron, M. & Volkow, N. (2007a). Effects of stimulant medication on growth rates across 3 years in the MTA follow-up. *Journal of the American Academy of Child and Adolescent Psychiatry, 46*, 1015–1027; Swanson, J., Hinshaw, S., Arnold, L., Gibbons, R., Marcus, S., Hur, K., Jensen, P., Vitiello, B., Abikoff, H., Greenhill, L., Hechtman, L., Pelham, W., Wells, K., Conners, C., March, J., Elliott, G., Epstein, J., Hoagwood, K., Hoza, B., Molina, B., Newcorn, J., Severe, J. & Wigal, T. (2007b). Second evaluation of MTA 36-month outcomes: Propensity score and growth mixture model analyses. *Journal of the American Academy of Child & Adolescent Psychiatry, 46*, 989–1002.
25. Aarskog, D., Fevang, F., Klove, H., Stoa, K., & Thorsen, T. (1977). The effect of stimulant drugs, dextroamphetamine and methylphenidate on secretion of growth hormone in hyperactive children. *Journal of Pediatrics, 90*, 136–139.
26. Firestone, P., Musten, L., Pisterman, S., Mercer, J. & Bennett, S. (1998). Short-term side effects of stimulant medication are increased in preschool children with attention-deficit/hyperactivity disorder: A double-blind placebo-controlled study. *Journal of Child & Adolescent Psychopharmacology, 8*, 13–25.

27. Mayes, S., Crites, D., Bixler, E. O., Humphrey, F. J. & Mattison, R. E. (1994). Methylphenidate and ADHD: Influence of age, IQ, and neurodevelopmental status. *Developmental Medicine and Child Neurology, 36*, 1099–1107.

28. Borcherding, B., Keysor, C., Rapoport, J., Elia, J. & Amass, J. (1990). Motor/vocal tics and compulsive behaviours on stimulant drugs: Is there a common vulnerability? *Psychiatric Research, 33*, 83–94.

29. Reviewed in Breggin, 2008b. See note 8.

30. Ibid., pp. 303–305; Moncrieff J. (2007b). Understanding psychotropic drug action: The contribution of the brain-disabling theory. *Ethical Human Psychology and Psychiatry, 9*, 170–179.

31. Breggin, 2008b. See note 8.

32. Swanson, J., Elliott, G., Greenhill, L., Wigal, T., Arnold, L., Vitiello, B., Hechtman, L., Epstein, J., Pelham, W., Abikoff, H., Newcorn, J., Molina, B., Hinshaw, S., Wells, K., Hoza, B., Jensen, P., Gibbons, R., Hur, K., Stehli, A., Davies, M., March, J., Conners, C., Caron, M. & Volkow, N. (2007). Effects of stimulant medication on growth rates across 3 years in the MTA follow-up. *Journal of the American Academy of Child and Adolescent Psychiatry, 46*, 1015–1027. 2007a. See note 24.

33. This section on stimulants was adapted from Breggin, P. (2013). *Psychiatric Drug Withdrawal: A guide for prescribers, therapists, patients and their families*. New York: Springer Publishing Company (which contains additional commentary and citations).

34. *Drug Facts and Comparisons* (2012). St. Louis, MO: Wolters Kluwer Health.

35. Chouinard, G. & Jones, B. (1980). Neuroleptic-induced supersensitivity psychosis: Clinical and pharmacologic characteristics. *American Journal of Psychiatry, 137*, 16–21. Reviewed in Breggin, 2008b, pp. 57–58. See note 8.

36. American Psychiatric Association (2000). *Diagnostic and Statistical Manual of Mental Disorders* (Fourth Edition, Text Revision). Washington, DC: APA, p. 803; Grohol, J. M. (2012). Final DSM-5 approved by American Psychiatric Association. Available at http://psychcentral.com/blog/archives/2012/12/02/final-dsm-5-approved-by-american-psychiatric-association/ (retrieved 13 February 2013).

37. Rosebush, P. & Mazurek, M. (1999). Neurologic side effects in neuroleptic-naïve patients treated with haloperidol or risperidone. *Neurology, 52*, 782–785; Lieberman, J., Stroup, T., McEvoy, J., Swartz, M., Rosenheck, R., Perkins, D., Keefe, R., Davis, S., Davis, C., Lebowitz, B., Severe. J. & Hsiao, J. (2005). Effectiveness of antipsychotic drugs in patients with chronic schizophrenia. *New England Journal of Medicine, 353*, 1209–1223.

38. Nasrallah, H. (2007). The roles of efficacy, safety, and tolerability in antipsychotic effectiveness: Practical implications of the CATIE schizophrenia trial. *Journal of Clinical Psychiatry, 68* (Suppl. 1) 5–11; Miller, R. (2009). Mechanisms of action of antipsychotic drugs of different classes, refractoriness to therapeutic effects of classical neuroleptics, and individual variation in sensitivity to their actions: Part II. *Current Neuropharmacology, 7*, 315–330.

39. Woods, S., Morgenstern, H., Saksa, J., Walsh, B., Sullivan, M., Money, R., Hawkins, K., Gueorguieva, R. & Glazer, W. (2010). Incidence of tardive dyskinesia with atypical versus conventional antipsychotic medication: A prospective cohort study. *Journal of Clinical Psychiatry, 71*, 463–474.

40. Reviewed in Breggin, 2008b, pp. 75–78. See note 8.

41. Breggin, P. (1979). *Psychiatric drugs: Hazards to the brain*. New York: Springer Publishing Company. See also Mejia, N. & Jankovic, J. (2010). Tardive dyskinesia and withdrawal emergent syndrome in children. *Expert Review of Neurotherapeutics, 10*, 893–901.

42. Reviewed in Breggin, P. (1990). Brain damage, dementia and persistent cognitive dysfunction associated with neuroleptic drugs: Evidence, etiology, implications. *Journal

of Mind and Behaviour, 11, 425–464; and Breggin, P. (1993). Parallels between neuroleptic effects and lethargic encephalitis: The production of dyskinesias and cognitive disorders. *Brain and Cognition*, 23, 8–27.

43. Ho, B.-C., Andreasen, N., Ziebell, S., Pierson, R. & Magnotta, V. (2011). Long-term antipsychotic treatment and brain volumes: A longitudinal study of first-episode schizophrenia. *Archives of General Psychiatry*, 68, 128–137; Levin, A. (2011). Brain volume shrinkage parallels rise in antipsychotic dosage. *Psychiatric News*, 8 May 2011, p. 1; van Haren, N., Schnack, H., Cahn, W., van den Heuvel, M., Lepage, C., Colloings, L., Evans, A., Pol, J. & Kahn, R. (2011). Changes in cortical thickness during the course of illness in schizophrenia. *Archives or General Psychiatry*, 68, 871–880.

44. Dorph-Petersen, K. A., Pierri, J., Perel, J., Sun, Z., Sampson, A. & Lewis, D. (2005). The influence of chronic exposure to antipsychotic medications on brain size before and after tissue fixation: A comparison of haloperidol and olanzapine in macaque monkeys. *Neuropsychopharmacology*, 30, 1649–1661; Konopaske, G., Dorph-Petersen, K. A., Pierri, J., Wu, Q., Sampson, A. & Lewis, A. (2007). Effect of chronic exposure to antipsychotic medication on cell numbers in the parietal cortex of macaque monkeys. *Neuropsychopharmacology*, 32, 1216–1223; Konopaske, G., Dorph-Petersen, K. A., Sweet, R., Pierri, J., Zhang, W., Sampson, A. & Lew, D. (2008). Effect of chronic antipsychotic exposure to astrocyte and oligodendrocytic numbers in macaque monkeys. *Biological Psychiatry*, 63, 759–765; Navari, S. & Dazzan, P. (2009). Do antipsychotic drugs affect brain structure? A systematic and critical review of MRI findings. *Psychological Medicine*, 39, 1763–1777.

45. Reviewed in Breggin, 2013. See note 33.

46. Gualtieri, C. & Barnhill, L. (1988). Tardive dyskinesia in special populations. In M. E. Wolf & A. D. Mosnaim (Eds). *Tardive Dyskinesia: Biological mechanisms and clinical aspects* (pp. 135–154). Washington, DC: American Psychiatric Press, p. 149; Myslobodsky, M. (1986). Anosognosia in tardive dyskinesia: 'Tardive dysmentia' or 'tardive dementia'? *Schizophrenia Bulletin*, 12, 1–6; Myslobodsky, M. (1993). Central determinants of attention and mood disorder in tardive dyskinesia ('tardive dysmentia'). *Brain and Cognition*, 23, 88–101.

47. See Breggin, 2008b. See note 8; Chouinard & Jones, 1980. See note 35; Moncrieff, J. (2006). Why is it so difficult to stop psychiatric treatment? It may be nothing to do with the original problem. *Medical Hypotheses*, 67, 517–523.

48. Gualtieri & Barnhill, 1988. See note 46.

49. Barnes, T. & McPhillips, M. (1995). How to distinguish between the neuroleptic-induced deficit syndrome, depression and disease-related negative symptoms in schizophrenia. *International Clinical Psychopharmacology*, 10 (Suppl. 3) 115–121.

50. Lieberman, J. & Stroup, T. (2011). The NIMH-CATIE schizophrenia study: What did we learn? *American Journal of Psychiatry*, 168, 770–775.

51. Splete, H. (2011). Antipsychotics linked to metabolic syndrome spike in children. *Clinical Psychiatry News*. Available at http://www.clinicalpsychiatrynews.com/single-view/antipsychotics-linked-to-metabolic-syndrome-spike-in-children/934df78c22.html (retrieved 11 September 2011); Goeb, J. L., Marco, S., Duhamel, A., Kechid, G., Bordet, R., Thomas, P., Delion, P. & Jardri, R. (2010). Metabolic side effects of risperidone in early onset schizophrenia. *Encephale*, 36, 242–252.

52. Moreno, C., Laje, G., Blanco, C., Jiang, H., Schmidt, A. & Olfson, M. (2007). National trends in the outpatient diagnosis and treatment of bipolar disorder in youth. *Archives of General Psychiatry*, 64, 1032–1039.

53. Sarchet, P. (2011). Harvard scientists disciplined for not declaring ties to drug companies. *Nature News Blog*, July 11. Available at http://blogs.nature.com/news/2011/07/Harvard_scientists_disciplined.html (retrieved 4 July 2011).

54. See, for example, Littrell, J. & Lyons, P. (2010a). Pediatric bipolar disorder: Part I – Is

it related to classical bipolar disorder? *Children and Youth Services Review, 32*, 965–973; Littrell, J. & Lyons, P. (2010b). Pediatric bipolar disorder: An issue for child welfare. *Children and Youth Services Review, 32*, 965–973.

55. Kilbourne, A., Ignacio, R., Kim, H. & Blow, F. (2009). Are VA patients with serious mental illness dying younger? *Psychiatric Services, 60*, 589; Parks, J., Svendsen, D., Singer, P., Foti, M. E. & Mauer, B. (2006). *Morbidity and Mortality in People with Serious Mental Illness*. Alexandria, VA: National Association of State Mental Health Program Directors. See the extensive review in Whitaker, R. (2010). *Anatomy of an Epidemic*. New York: Crown.

56. Sundell, K., Gissler, M., Petzold, M. & Waern, M. (2011). Antidepressant utilization patterns and mortality in Swedish men and women aged 20–34 years. *European Journal of Clinical Pharmacology, 67*, 169–178.

57. Joukamaa, M., Heliovaara, M., Knekt, P., Aromaa, A., Raitasalo, R. & Lehtinen, V. (2006). Schizophrenia, neuroleptic medication and mortality. *British Journal of Psychiatry, 188*, 122–127. See also Gill, S., Bronskill, S., Normand, S. L., Anderson, M., Sykora, K., Lam, K., Bell, C., Lee, P., Fischer, H., Herrmann, N., Gurwitz, J. & Rochon, P. (2007). Antipsychotic drug use and mortality in older adults with dementia. *Annals of Internal Medicine, 146*, 775–786; Dwyer, D., Lu, X. H. & Bradley, J. (2003). Cytotoxicity of conventional and atypical antipsychotic drugs in relation to glucose metabolism. *Brain Research, 971*, 31–39.

58. Breggin, 2008b, Chapter Two. See note 8.

59. See note 44.

60. Lieberman et al, 2005, p. 1218. See note 37.

61. Lieberman & Stroup, 2011, p. 774. See note 50.

62. Ibid. p. 773.

63. For a review see Whitaker, R. (2010). *Anatomy of an Epidemic*. New York: Crown, pp. 99–104. An excellent overview of the problems associated with giving antipsychotic drugs to children can be found in: Whitaker, R. (2012). Weighing the evidence: What science has to say about prescribing atypical antipsychotics to children. In S. Olfman & B. Robbins (Eds). *Drugging our Children: How profiteers are pushing antipsychotics on our youngest and what we can do to stop it* (pp. 13–16). Santa Barbara, CA: Praeger.

64. This section on antipsychotic drugs, like the previous one on ADHD and stimulants, was adapted from Breggin, P. (2013). *Psychiatric Drug Withdrawal*. New York: Springer Publishing Company (which contains additional commentary and citations).

65. See Breggin, P. (1973). Psychosurgery. *Journal of the American Medical Association, 226*, 1121; Breggin, P. (1975). Psychosurgery for political purposes. *Duquesne Law Review, 13*, 841–862; Breggin, P. (1977). If psychosurgery is wrong in principle? *Psychiatric Opinion*, Nov–Dec, p. 23; Breggin, P. (1980). Brain-disabling therapies. In E. Valenstein (Ed.). *The Psychosurgery Debate*. San Francisco: W. H. Freeman; Breggin, P. (1981). Psychosurgery as brain-disabling treatments. In M. Dongier & D. Wittkower (Eds). *Divergent Views in Psychiatry* (pp. 302–326). Hagerstown, MD: Harper & Row.

66. Kaimowitz v. Department of Mental Health for the State of Michigan. 1973. No 73-19434-AW (Mich. Cir. Ct. Wayne County, July 10, 1973). Available at http://bit.ly/1NSO4b4 (retrieved 18 June 2015). Discussed in Breggin, 1975. See note 65.

67. Breggin, 2008b. See note 8.

68. Breggin, P. (2011). Psychiatric drug-induced chronic brain impairment (CBI): Implications for long-term treatment with psychiatric medication. *International Journal of Risk & Safety in Medicine, 23*, 193–200; Breggin, 2013. See note 33.

69. Gottstein, 2012. See note 1.

70. Breggin, P. (1991) *Toxic Psychiatry*. New York: St Martin's Press.

71. Breggin, 2013. See note 33.

Chapter 8

'Learning-disabled children'

Katherine Runswick-Cole
and Dan Goodley

In this chapter, we focus on the lives of 'learning-disabled children'. Our concern is to explore the ways in which the category of 'learning-disabled child' is produced and sustained in contemporary social and cultural contexts in England. These contexts include a host of social care, health and educational places as well as community settings. Crucially, we consider the impact of the category on children so labelled, and their families and allies. In exploring the category of 'learning-disabled child', we draw on our research collaborations with children, young people and their families over the past 10 years by drawing on findings from the authors' engagement with three research projects.[1]

To begin, we consider the categories 'learning disability' and 'child' in turn, before considering how the categories interconnect and intersect with one another. Next we consider the ways in which the category 'learning-disabled child' impacts on children's lives, drawing on examples from our research and focusing on the practices, systems and sites in which the category is reproduced, including the contexts of health, education and care. We argue that the concept of 'learning-disabled child', despite attempts to shake it off, is a sticky category that demands us to interrogate its often-disabling impacts on the lives of children and their families and allies. Whilst labels are a useful administrative category for accessing services and support, we seek to trouble their pathological tendencies. Our analysis is driven by the eclectic pulse of critical disability studies: an interdisciplinary community of theory, politics and activism that seeks to understand and trouble the precarious societal position held by disabled people. One key disciplinary approach is that of critical psychological disabilities, where we bring in perspectives such as social constructionism, discourse analysis and psycho-politics to understand the constitution of subjectivity, relationality and personhood as products of a (disabling) world.[2] We conclude that 'learning-disabled children' are not passive beings merely acted upon, but rather that they are full of potential and have the capacity to reshape, refashion and revise the normative expectations that cloud their lives in ways which impact positively on their lives and, indeed, all children's lives.

Learning disability

From the beginning, we have to acknowledge that, from the latter part of the twentieth century onwards, academics have played a significant part in both producing and sustaining the category of 'learning disability'. We agree with Carlson that the proliferation of the category 'learning disability' has been enabled by a rise in the number of new techniques and technologies that are used to gather information about people.[3] The category has also kept a fair few professionals in work, including psychologists. We know too that the production of the category 'learning disability' by the academic community has and continues to provide legitimisation of the institutionalisation and oppression of disabled people. It is important to recognise, then, that labels are and always have been contentious; while they have been used in enabling ways in children's lives to gain access to services and support, they can simultaneously threaten and limit people's lives.[4] In engaging with a discussion of the category of the 'learning-disabled child' our aim is not to contribute to the maintenance of what we would see as a potentially oppressive and disabling category, but to trouble, reshape and revise it in order to promote more enabling understandings of the category which will impact positively on the lives of the people who are touched by it. We acknowledge that learning disability exists but we often wonder why.

'Learning disability' is only one of a cluster of labels that has been used to refer to 'lack of intelligence'. Across the globe, the terms 'mental handicap', 'retardation', 'intellectual disability', 'cognitive impairment' and 'developmental delay' are in widespread use.[5] These terms are all premised on individualistic and medicalised understandings of 'learning disability' that locate the 'problem' within a person 'with a learning disability' with the firm belief that the cause of any difficulty is to be found in the realm of biomedicine.[6] In 1982 Bogdan and Taylor mounted a blistering attack on bi-medical and psychological understandings of learning disability:

> Mental retardation [sic] is, in fact, a socio-political not a psychological construction. The myth, perpetuated by a society which refuses to recognise the true nature of its needed social reforms, has successfully camouflaged the politics of diagnosis and incarceration.[7]

Despite this and other concerted attempts to shift understandings and to explore the discursive and socially constructed nature of the concept of 'learning disability', official definitions in England still draw on individual and medicalised approaches.[8] So, for instance, the *Valuing People* white paper, a policy document which set out the New Labour government's strategy for learning disability for the twenty-first century (and was then taken up by the Conservative–Liberal Democrat Coalition government in the UK), still holds onto the following definition:

> Learning disability includes the presence of:
> - A significantly reduced ability to understand new or complex information, to learn new skills (impaired intelligence), with:
> - A reduced ability to cope independently (impaired social functioning);
> - Which started before adulthood, with a lasting effect on development.[9]

For some readers of this volume, our claims for a social constructionist account of the category of 'learning disability' will simply seem as if we are arguing against the commonsensical importance of labelling. Labels are useful, aren't they? Moreover, learning disabilities are a reality for some children? This response is not surprising; in contemporary global-North contexts people labelled with learning disabilities have been de-culturised – they are positioned as lacking, alone and as 'other'.[10] Learning disability is still widely understood as a 'naturalised impairment' beyond the realm or reach of the social.[11] Contemporary discourses of neuroscience tantalisingly promise, but have so far failed to deliver, a 'real' account of the causes and aetiology of learning disability and yet this is a promise to which we, in contemporary global-North cultures, remain optimistically attached.[12] Despite this persistent attachment to a naturalised category of learning disability, not all seemingly 'natural' categories have been so resistant to a social constructionist critique; indeed, one example of a category that has been shaped by this critique is the category 'child'.

Children and childhood

Childhood has also been widely understood as a naturalised category (see, Chapter 1, this volume). And yet, more recently, understandings of the concepts of children and childhood as being socially constructed are broadly accepted within the academy in the global North. For example, James and Prout argue that 'childhood' is a social phenomenon that can never be separated from other variables such as class, gender or ethnicity.[13] In 1962 Ariès published a hugely influential text, *Centuries of Childhood*, in which he argued that, although 'childhood' is often presented as a natural phenomenon, 'childhood' simply did not exist in the Medieval era as infancy and adulthood were distinguished without an intervening period of childhood being acknowledged.[14] The shifting focus on children as 'active social agents' within childhood studies represents a further change in how 'child' is reproduced and reconstructed.[15] The impact of the deconstruction of the naturalised child and the reconstruction of the child as an agent in the social world has been far reaching. In both UK national and international law children's rights have been asserted.[16] And yet, while the idea of the child as a social construction has been largely accepted in relations to class, gender or ethnicity, disability is usually missing from the mix. While norms associated with class, gender and ethnicity are frequently troubled within childhood studies, a continued attachment to notions of 'normal' child development means that learning disability remains firmly within the realm of the 'natural'.

The 'learning-disabled child'

From the beginning of a baby's life (and sometimes before) the 'hunt' for learning disability is on and, make no mistake, this is an urgent search.[17] The practices of early identification promise rehabilitation and cure, but only if you intervene early enough. Ever-increasingly narrow definitions of the 'normal' child circulate as the number of labels for children who differ from the 'norm' increase, including: attention deficit hyperactivity disorder (ADHD), oppositional defiance disorder (ODD), and deficits in attention, motor control and perception (DAMP), among many others.[18]

At the same time, 'learning-disabled people' are still characterised as being in some ways 'childlike', and as behaving like or having the same cognitive abilities as a child. In England this childlike status has been reinforced by the introduction of Education, Health and Care plans which chart progress and support needs from birth to 25.[19]

This conflation of 'learning disabled' and 'childlike' has had devastating consequences on the lives of 'learning-disabled people' who have been denied the right to vote, love, have sex, have children, work and to make choices about where they live and whom they live with. Moreover, it is especially difficult to get away with pastimes such as drug taking, alcohol use and partying if you have the label of learning disability.

Despite attempts, with varying degrees of success, to trouble both the category of the 'learning disabled' and 'child' outlined above, the 'learning-disabled child' persists as a naturalised entity in policy and practice in England. For example, recent education and health policy reiterates the understanding of learning disability as a within-child deficit:

> A child of compulsory school age or a young person has a learning difficulty or disability if he or she:
> - has a significantly greater difficulty in learning than the majority of others of the same age, or
> - has a disability which prevents or hinders him or her from making use of facilities of a kind generally provided for others of the same age in mainstream schools or mainstream post-16 institutions.[20]

So far we have sought to unsettle in the category 'learning-disabled child' but we acknowledge that the category persists in policy and practice in England. In what follows, we return to three research projects, drawing on stories from the lives of 'learning-disabled' children and young people, as well as from their families and allies, to explore how this sticky and persistent category impacts on everyday lives.

The research projects

This chapter draws on the insights gained from three research projects through which we have engaged with the lives of 'learning-disabled' children and young people over the last 10 years. We describe each of these projects in turn.

1. Parents, professionals and disabled babies: Identifying enabling care, 2003–2006

This ESRC-funded study was undertaken collaboratively by the University of Sheffield and Newcastle University in the UK from 2003 to 2006. The research aimed to identify principles of enabling care from the perspectives of parents of disabled babies and allied professionals.[21]

In-depth interviews were conducted with 25 families with babies and young children with special care needs. There was also a strong ethnographic component to the methodology, involving: (i) the observation of mothers, children and professionals in a variety of clinical, social services and social-service and home settings; and (ii) immersion within the wider support networks of parents. Finally, focus groups were carried out to include the perspectives of a range of medical and social care professionals working with the families.[22]

2. Does every child matter, post-Blair?
The interconnections of disabled childhoods, 2008–2011[23]

This project was based at Manchester Metropolitan University, in collaboration with Newcastle University. The aim of the project was to understand what it meant to be a disabled child growing up in England. The study was based in the north of England and ran from September 2008 to April 2011. The participants included disabled children aged four to 16, their parents/carers and professionals who work with disabled children, including teachers, third sector workers, health workers and social workers. Data collection included interviews using multimedia methods. The interviews were open-ended and covered a range of issues, including children and young people's experiences of health, social care, education and leisure. A period of ethnography involved attending children's birthday parties, bowling, shopping with families, as well as attending impairment-specific leisure activities, including an autism-specific social club, parent groups, and user consultation meetings set up by local authorities, services and professionals to access the views of families. Finally, the research also included focus group interviews with professionals ranging from teachers and social workers to speech pathologists, advocates, and leisure providers.[24]

3. Big Society? Disabled people with learning disabilities and civil society, 2013–2015

The project ran from June 2013 to June 2015 as a partnership between four universities (Manchester Metropolitan University, the University of Sheffield, the University of Bristol and Northumbria University) working with partner organisations in the UK (Speakup Self Advocacy, the Foundation for People with Learning Disabilities, Mencap, Manchester Learning Disability Partnership, Pathways Associates and independent living consultants). The overall research question asked: How are disabled people with learning disabilities faring in

Big Society? The research was carried out through seven overlapping and interconnected phases, including interviews and ethnographic encounters.[25]

The 'learning-disabled child' emerges

In what follows, we explore the processes and practices in which the 'learning-disabled child' emerges. Following our rejection of the category of 'learning-disabled child' as 'natural', we explore the encounters, moments, systems and sites in which the 'learning-disabled child' is made, and ask what impact this has on the child and those around them. We begin at one of the moments when the 'learning-disabled child' first appears: the point of diagnosis.

Diagnosis

> You know, when you go for an assessment and they ask you all these questions, it was only at that point that I thought, 'Oh, okay, that's considered bizarre behaviour.' I didn't realise that. (Gayle, mother, Study 2)[26]

Gayle recalls the moment that her son was given his first diagnosis: attention deficit hyperactivity disorder (ADHD). By the age of seven, Simon had been labelled in turn as 'normal', 'naughty', 'having ADHD' and finally as having 'Asperger syndrome and dyspraxia'. Gayle described the positive effects of labelling: a label gave her access to Disability Living Allowance (state benefits in England), to a Statement of Special Educational Needs (setting out the extra provision her son would need in school), and to an ADHD nurse (a specialist nurse to support Gayle in managing her son's behaviour). Clearly, some diagnostic labels can function as powerful markers that provide a passport to services and support. Gill (a mother, Study 1) explained how a label helped her explain her child to her family: 'But it's just the way people are; I think they prefer it when there is a label attached because then they can deal with it a lot easier, I mean, especially the family.'

The consequences for Simon of the emergence as a 'learning-disabled child' were far-reaching. His feelings of anger became 'autistic meltdowns'; riding a bike was 'part of his physiotherapy programme to strengthen his core stability'; and going to bed became part of a 'structured approach to behaviour management'.[27] It felt as if Simon, the 'learning-disabled child', had become known and could only be known through the diagnostic labels that engulfed him and his family.

While the 'learning-disabled child' often emerges at the point of diagnosis, glimpses of 'difference and disorder' are often visible before diagnosis in a variety of different cultural contexts and practices. Medical diagnosis in young children often occurs as a process rather than a one-off event. For Gayle, diagnosis offered a moment of realisation, but this was inevitably preceded by a period of assessment in which Simon was measured against the 'norm' and found to be an unacceptable distance from it. The hunting grounds for difference occupy many and varied terrains in education and in health but sites for children's play have traditionally presented an open space with an unimpeded view for those in search of the 'learning-disabled child'.

Play

Spaces for play, it seems, afford rich pickings for the practices of assessment and categorisation of learning disability, offering potentially rich pickings. 'Learning-disabled children's' play is characterised as both different and deficient in comparison with their 'non-disabled' peers. Play is monitored, surveilled and managed through the discourses of impairment. Play can be 'good' (typical) or 'bad' (atypical and disordered). And so, flapping your arms or waving your fingers in front of your eyes is a red flag for autism;[28] parallel play (beyond an 'appropriate' age) a sign of 'developmental delay'.[29] Sarah recalls a painful encounter between her daughter, Chrissie, and a playworker intent on making Chrissie play 'appropriately':

> The thing that didn't work was [the playworker] trying to make her do pretend play. No, she is really not interested in giving a drink to the dolly, she has no interest in dollies! NO, NO, this is not, NOT working! (Sarah, Study 2)[30]

As Sarah's story reveals above, play, for the 'learning-disabled child', becomes a site for identification and intervention as well as a site of construction of the category. The shift from play to rehabilitation has consequences for the child and those around them. Lynne described the playworker coming to her house and feeling that her abilities were being questioned:

> It seemed as if they [the playworker] were coming [to the home] for no reason ... they were told to come to somebody's house and show this family how to play with this [child] and we knew that ... we knew how to

> show him how to push a car along. You know, 'Come on Robert, let's play cars,' or 'Let's play in the sandpit.' (Lynne, mother, Study 2)[31]

Once a 'learning-disabled child' has been identified, both they and their primary carer (usually the mother) are considered to be in deficit and lack; they become subjects of surveillance and intervention.

Education

In England early education is premised on the mantra of 'learning through play'; in the early years, at least, play is undeniably the child's work.[32] In failing to play 'appropriately' and failing to respond to the urgent interventions of practitioners in the early years, the 'learning-disabled child' is remade, yet again, in the context of more formal education. A 1970 report from the President's Committee on Mental Retardation entitled *The Six-hour Mentally Retarded Child* describes how a whole host of children were defined as 'retarded children' solely between the hours of 9.00am and 4.00pm, five days a week, and yet the naturalised category 'learning-disabled child' remains intact in schools.[33]

In England the 'learning-disabled child' is not only at significantly higher risk of exclusion than 'non-disabled' peers, but he or she is also constructed as posing a significant threat to the economic progress of the wider community.[34] Since 1997 successive governments' educational policy has called for the assimilation of 'learning-disabled children'. The previous UK Conservative–Liberal Democrat Coalition government asserted that: '[i]f more effective support of disabled children and children with SEN [special educational needs] prompted greater achievement, it could result in higher productivity gains and growth for the economy, thereby benefiting both the individual and society.'[35] 'Learning-disabled children' are, then, characterised as a threat to themselves, their family and to a productive society.[36]

Schools produce and sustain the category of the 'learning-disabled child'. They not only play their part in the assessment and diagnostic process that identifies children whose lack of achievement, we are told, threatens the individual child and the wider society; but also they engage in a host of practices that mark the child as different from their peers, as this encounter reveals:

> Kamil wanders around the room not involved in the painting activity; eventually he decides to join in the activity and sits down to take a paintbrush. The teaching assistant takes it out of his hand (there is a

minor struggle) and says 'paint finished' and gives him a coloured pencil instead. He loses interest and leaves the table again and begins to wander about the classroom. (Katherine's ethnographic notes, Study 2)[37]

In wandering round the room, Kamil fails to conform to expected classroom norms. In response to his non-compliance, he is punished: 'paint finished' and is left to occupy the margins of the classroom, yet again. Parents and carers also described the very public ways in which 'learning-disabled children' were physically marked as different in schools:

I'd seen in nursery in that Andrew was dragged by the hand into the hall, sat down and it was just like 'the naughty child' really. I felt as a parent I wanted to be in there saying, 'Don't do that to my child.' You expect that people in educational establishments and with that sort of training wouldn't be doing these kinds of things and again, from a parent's perspective, you don't always feel comfortable with going in all the time, because you know you are classified as the parent who is always ... (Lucy, mother, Study 2)[38]

In our work in schools, we found that 'learning-disabled children' were often physically separated from their 'non-disabled peers': in different rooms for lunch, in separate spaces in the playground and in 'special' classrooms or units in their 'mainstream' schools. This physical separation was reinforced with the kinds of practices experienced by Kamil and Andrew alongside discursive repertoires that frame 'learning-disabled children' as 'other', describing 'them' as 'the special needs', deprived of their status as child.[39] While we accept the need for schools to be safe places, we see an irony in the unruly acts of practitioners (grabbing arms and hands) being offered as evidence of the child's difference and disorder.

'Learning-disabled children' are made by and subjected to the (grim) practical realities of schooling. Schools are 'highly stressful' systems: schools are subjected to league tables, teachers to inspection, and children to constant assessment and testing. Elsewhere we have described the ways in which such stressful school environments produce systemic violence against 'learning-disabled children'.[40] Drawing on Žižek's notion of systemic violence, which views violence as part of the maintenance of the system, the marking and manhandling of 'learning-disabled children' in schools can be seen as a direct product of the system. It is a system that requires regulation, governance and control. It is not surprising, then, that educational professionals 'do these kinds of things' and 'use that kind of language', because they find themselves acting in such ways to fit the rigidity of the system.

Violence and 'learning-disabled children'

Sadly, however, it is the image of 'learning-disabled children' as a violent threat that is the well-worn cultural trope in the global North. Take, for example, two stories from our research:

> It's finding the people [to look after him] that could actually physically cope with my son. Because if he doesn't co-operate, you have to manhandle him, to get him out of the door and, you know, he'll be punching you, kicking you. (Roberta, mother, Study 2)[41]

> My daughter has a good line in hand-biting and hitting people which really upsets the escort on the minibus. I think at some point, if she actually manages to get the escort, I think he'll say, 'I'm not having that child on my bus ever again.' (Shelley, mother, Study 2)[42]

These accounts appear to support the idea that violence and 'learning-disabled children' are inextricably connected; they are enmeshed to create a pathological whole. That the version of the 'learning-disabled child' as 'mad' or 'bad' dominates is a testimony to the extensive reaches of a learning-disability discourse that perpetuates the myth of naturalised deficit and disorder in children.

Far from being the pathological perpetrators of violence, we found that 'learning-disabled children' were more likely to be the victims of violence, not only in schools, but in their local communities:

> She got bullied by girls on the school bus; they pinned her down and were putting tampons in her mouth ... We stuck it out on the bus a bit longer and then I thought no, so that's why we give her the lift. (Lesley, mother, Study 2)[43]

> Because the thing that we've had with his school now, they don't tell any staff, he's actually been physically assaulted by a lunchtime supervisor. She thought he'd been bullying her granddaughter, she hit him in the dining hall and said she'd 'bloody kill him' next time. (Gayle, mother, Study 2)[44]

> The youth worker called me into her office. She looked dreadful, shocked. Eventually she told me that there had been an incident in the toilet. A

group of girls had been teasing Isobel and they tried to get her to lick the toilet seat. There was a rumour that the whole thing had been videoed on a camera-phone and posted on YouTube. (Alex, mother, Study 2)[45]

These accounts confirm that the 'learning-disabled child' is often the victim of violence by 'non-disabled' others. When confronted with such stories, we know that there is a temptation to respond to these accounts of violence as the actions of 'a few bad people'. Our concern is that blaming a few individuals detracts attention from the discursive and cultural conditions that produce environments in which violence against 'learning-disabled children' becomes almost a mundane, everyday occurrence. Our focus should be on those conditions of institutionalised violence and systemic failure that perpetuate threats to the lives of people associated with the label of learning disabilities.

Death

So far, we have argued that almost every aspect of the 'learning-disabled child's' life is subjected to scrutiny and surveillance. We have described the ways in which urgent and early intervention is prescribed in 'learning-disabled children's' lives to ensure that their development can be as close to the (mythical) norm as possible. We have shown how, in schools, the 'learning-disabled child' becomes subject to the pressures of a system that demands certain forms of performance and achievement, and how failure to live up to these expectations results in violence in schools and in wider communities.

There is one area of the 'learning-disabled child's' life that has received much less interest or scrutiny, and that is death. Relatively little is known about the lives of disabled children who are dying. Todd concluded that this lack of interest unwittingly conveys a sense that the death of a disabled child is in some way less important than other deaths. Parents of disabled children who die young report the discrimination they face as their grief is seen as an illegitimate response to their child's death.[46] The death of a 'learning-disabled child' is seen by those around them as a release from what is perceived to be the overwhelmingly negative experience of parenting a disabled child.[47]

The different cultural status of the death of a 'learning-disabled child' is revealed in the fact that the sudden and unexpected deaths of 'learning-disabled children and young people' often go unreported in the media. Ryan describes how it took eight months and a campaign on social media before the mainstream media reported the death of her son, Connor, a young 'learning-disabled man', who died in the care of the National Health Service in England.[48] Connor, who also had epilepsy, drowned, unsupervised, in the bath; an independent review found his death to be preventable. And yet Ryan described how, for eight months, she had watched as other young people's sudden and tragic deaths were reported immediately. When an English backpacker on a gap year between school and university dies, the media reports this the next day. The young backpacker is described in reference to an imagined future as, perhaps, a doctor, a lawyer or a teacher. In contrast, the reports of Connor's death made no mention of the life he might have had, leaving Ryan to conclude that there are no imagined futures for young 'learning-disabled people'. Characterised as being in deficit and lack, and as threatening, rather than contributing to, the future of the economy and social cohesion, 'learning-disabled children and young people' experience discrimination, not only in life but in death.

Possibilities for resistance and a politics for change

While being careful not to deny or devalue the often difficult and painful experiences of the 'learning-disabled children' we have worked with, we do also see possibilities for resistance and the potential of a politics for change in 'learning-disabled children's' lives. The politicisation of the lives of disabled children has gathered momentum, in part, we hope, through empirical and theoretical work associated within our disciplinary home, critical disability studies. We argue that 'learning-disabled children' are full of potential: they have potential to subvert, rethink and reject narrow, dull, normative, limiting, disabling, conservative and exclusionary practices in schools, their communities and in wider society. 'Learning-disabled children' transgress normal and normative ways of life and demand those allied with them to do the same.

'Learning-disabled children' and their allies

The potential for 'learning-disabled children' and their allies to transgress the normative in positive and enabling ways was clearly demonstrated by the children and young people we worked with. We share three examples here to illustrate our findings: queer schools, participation in the arts, and circles of support.

Crip schools

> Northtown is a co-located special school. Both the head teacher of Northtown and the mainstream school head were keen to co-locate.

> They both saw this as an opportunity for inclusion but also saw the potential that sharing resources might have for improving provision for both schools. The schools share the sports facilities, canteen, school hall and theatre. The schools share one reception area but the special school is on one half of the building and the mainstream school on the other ... There had been concerns that the mainstream pupils would tease or stare at or name-call the disabled pupils but this hasn't happened ... The school itself is extremely well appointed with breakout areas, interactive whiteboards, a sensory room, huge accessible changing/toilet facilities, music, art, science rooms and soft play. The atmosphere in the school was incredibly calm and purposeful with children engaged in a range of practical activities. The art room was stunning and I met the art teacher who the Deputy Head had described as 'bonkers' but brilliant. This seemed to be a bit of a theme among the staff. The science teacher was constructing a display that would use lighting to move from day to night and different creatures would emerge throughout the day. This was alongside his construction of a display that glows under UV lights. He uses projectors to display moving pictures of animals and UV paint to bring to life a huge ant ... The Deputy Head said that the science teachers visiting from the mainstream school had said, 'Why can't we teach science like this?' (Ethnographic notes, Study 2)[49]

In exploring these practices we have drawn on the tools of queer and crip theory. We see the 'bonkers' teacher as a queer teacher, someone who is prepared to take risks. The queer teacher responds to the queer children in his/her class with an inclusive and creative approach, offering opportunities for what McKenzie terms *possability*: the ways in which 'learning-disabled children' demand imaginative and responsive forms of educational provision.[50] Normative teaching is narrow, competitive, dull; queer teaching is guided by creative pedagogies, wonder, quirkiness and difference. Queer teaching is a response to queer children ('learning-disabled children') that demands more imaginative approaches to teaching and learning for all.

Participation in the arts

Participation in the arts also offers a space to celebrate wonder, inclusivity and quirkiness. However, where disabled children's participation in the arts has been the focus of research, this has often been limited to an evaluation of the impact of rehabilitation through drama therapy on 'learning-disabled children's' lives.[51] Participation in the arts has been another site of construction of and rehabilitation of the 'learning-disabled child'. In our work with children and young people, we found examples of performance being used to support the personal and sociopolitical development of disabled young people. We found that participation in the arts can promote 'learning-disabled children's' wellbeing and their sense of belonging. We found that performance allowed for diverse ways of being, of playing and of learning.[52]

In our work with the Oily Cart theatre company we found that perceptions of 'learning-disabled children' were changed through their participation in the arts, as one person commented as she entered the theatre: 'This [performance] shows that they ['learning-disabled children'] matter and that somebody cares and somebody has invested' (Mother, Study 2). A teacher felt that through engagement with the performance, she would seek to be more playful in her work in the classroom.[53] Through participation in the arts 'learning-disabled children' were able to shake off their sticky label, if only temporarily, and to reclaim their status as childlike and playful without reference to the shadow of the norm.[54]

Networks and communities

> We're in transition – that horrible halfway space between children's and adults' services, a no man's land littered with the complex policies and procedures of health, education and social care.
>
> My son Henry is 17; he is much loved and loving; he enjoys pylons, parsnip crisps and chocolate as well as his computer; he has an eclectic taste in music ranging from Aha and Duran Duran to Ellie Goulding. He is great company out on a walk or going to the shops, and, over the years, he has also collected a range of labels including 'having a learning disability'. (Henry's mum, Study 3)

In a series of blog posts Henry's mum (pseudonym) describes bringing together a circle of support around Henry to help her plan for his transition from child to adult services and from school to beyond.[55] In her accounts of the circle meeting, Henry's mum describes how a group of friends came together to support her and Henry to plan for the future. Her discussion is of Henry's interests and aspirations, activities and pastimes, hopes and dreams. We know from her first post that Henry has a 'learning disability' but in the subsequent blog posts Henry's label is absent. Symptoms, signs, diagnoses and prognosis are usurped by a focus on participation, aspiration, love and community. Through engagement with others who care for and about him, Henry has been able to remove the label of 'learning disability' and to focus on his hopes, dreams and aspirations.

Conclusion

In this chapter we have explored the category 'learning-disabled child' in contemporary social and cultural contexts in England. Drawing on three research projects in which we have worked alongside 'learning-disabled children and young people', we have explored the impact of the category on children's lives in their experiences of play, education, violence and death. While our accounts demonstrate the disabling effects of the persistently sticky category of the 'learning-disabled child', we have also explored the ways in which children and young people can resist, reshape and revise the category and demonstrate their potential in schools, participation in the arts and in their communities. We remain optimistic that 'learning-disabled children' may be able to peel off their sticky label and become, as Haraldsdóttir says, 'simply children'.[56] But we also recognise the ubiquitous signifier of 'learning disability' and seek to contest the associated signified meanings of lack, deficit and pathology.

Acknowledgements

We should like to thank the Economic and Social Research Council for their support and for funding each of the research projects we draw on in this chapter: Parents, professionals and disabled babies: Identifying enabling care (RES-000-23-0129); Does every child matter, post-Blair? The interconnections of disabled childhoods (RES-062-23-1138); Big Society? Disabled people with learning disabilities and civil society (RES/K004883/1).

Endnotes

1. a) Economic and Social Research Council (Grant No. RES-000-23-0129). Parents, professionals and disabled babies: Identifying enabling care (University of Sheffield) 2003–2006: This project asked what enabling care might look like for disabled babies and very young children. b) Economic and Social Research Council (Grant No. RES-062-23-1138). Does every child matter, post-Blair? The interconnections of disabled childhoods, 2008–2011 (see http://doeseverychildmatterpostblair.wordpress.com): This project asked what impact the changes in policy and practice for children in England since 1997 had had on the lives of disabled children and young people. c) Economic and Social Research Council (Grant No. ES/K004883/1) Big Society?

Disabled people with learning disabilities and civil society, 2013-2015 (see http://bigsocietydis.wordpress.com): This project explores how young people and adults with the label of learning disability are faring in the context of economic austerity in England and the extent to which they are participating in civil society.

2. For an overview see Goodley, D. (2010). *Disability Studies: An interdisciplinary introduction*. London: Sage.
3. Carlson, L. (2010). *The Faces of Intellectual Disability: Philosophical reflections*. Bloomington, IN: Indiana University Press.
4. Goodley, D. & Runswick-Cole, K. (2014a). Big Society? Disabled people with the label of learning disabilities and the queer(y)ing of civil society. *Scandinavian Journal of Disability Research, 17*, 1-13.
5. Ibid.; Goodley, D. & Runswick-Cole, K. (2014b). Critical psychologies of disability: Boundaries, borders and bodies in the lives of disabled children. *Emotional and Behavioural Difficulties, 20*, 51-63.
6. Oliver, M. (1990). *The Politics of Disablement*. Basingstoke: Macmillan.
7. Bogdan, R. & Taylor, S. J. (1982). *Inside Out: The social meaning of retardation*. Toronto: University of Toronto Press, p. 15.
8. Goodley, D. (2010). *Disability Studies: An interdisciplinary introduction*, London: Sage; Rapley, M. (2004). *The Social Construction of Intellectual Disability*. Cambridge: Cambridge University Press; Chapell, A. L. (1998). Still out in the cold: People with learning difficulties and the social model of disability. In T. Shakespeare (Ed.). *The Disability Reader: Social science perspectives*. London: Cassell.
9. Department of Health (2001). *Valuing People: A new strategy for learning disability for the 21st century*. London: Department of Health, p. 14.
10. Goodley, D. (2001). 'Learning difficulties', the social model of disability and impairment: Challenging epistemologies. *Disability and Society, 16* (2) 207-231.
11. Ibid.
12. Berlant, L. (2006). Cruel optimism. *Differences: A journal of feminist cultural studies, 17* (3) 20-36.
13. James, A. & Prout, J. (2001). *Constructing and Reconstructing Childhood: Contemporary issues in the sociological study of childhood*. London: Routledge.
14. Ariès, P. (1962). *Centuries of Childhood*. London: Cape Baker, 2002.
15. Mallett, R. & Runswick-Cole, K. (2014). *Approaching Disability: Critical issues and perspectives*. Abingdon: Routledge.
16. HMSO (1989). *The Children Act*. London: HMSO; UNICEF (1989). *UN Convention on the Rights of the Child*. Geneva: Office of the High Commissioner for Human Rights.
17. Baker, B. (2002). The hunt for disability: Eugenics and the normalization of school children. *Teachers College Record, 104* (4) 663-703, p. 663.
18. Goodley, 2010. See note 8.
19. Department for Education & Department for Health (2014). *Special Educational Needs and Disability Code of Practice: 0 to 25 years*. Available at https://www.gov.uk/government/uploads/system/uploads/attachment_data/file/342440/SEND_Code_of_Practice_approved_by_Parliament_29.07.14.pdf (retrieved May 2015).
20. Ibid. pp. 15-16.
21. McLaughlin, J., Goodley, D., Clavering, E. & Fisher, P. (2008). *Families Raising Disabled Children: Enabling care and social justice*. Basingstoke: Palgrave-Macmillan.
22. Fisher, P. & Goodley, D. (2007). The linear medical model of disability: Mothers of disabled babies resist with counter-narratives. *Sociology of Health & Illness, 29* (1) 66-81.
23. http://www.rihsc.mmu.ac.uk/postblairproject/

24. See ESRC (n.d.). Does every child matter, post Blair? The interconnections of disabled childhoods. Available at http://www.esrc.ac.uk/my-esrc/grants/res-062-23-1138/read (retrieved May 2015). Adapted from Goodley, D. & Runswick-Cole, K. (2010). Emancipating play: Dis/abled children, development and deconstruction. *Disability & Society,* 25 (4) 499–512.
25. More details available at http://bigsocietydis.wordpress.com/
26. Goodley, D. & Runswick-Cole, K. (2011a). Parents, professionals and disabled children: Exploring processes of dis/ablism. In L. O'Dell & S. Leverett (Eds). *Working with Children and Young People: Co-constructing practice.* Buckingham: Open University, p. 74.
27. Ibid. p. 75.
28. McGuire, A. (2011). Representing autism: A critical examination of autism advocacy in the neoliberal West. Unpublished PhD thesis, University of Toronto.
29. Goodley, D. & Runswick-Cole, K. (2010a) Emancipating play: Dis/abled children, development and deconstruction. *Disability & Society,* 25 (4) 499–512.
30. Ibid. p. 505.
31. Ibid.
32. Brodin, J. (2005). Diversity of aspects on play in children with profound multiple disabilities. *Early Child Development and Care,* 175 (17) 635–646.
33. Langness, L. L. & Levine, H. G. (Eds) (1986). *Culture and Retardation: Life histories of mildly mentally retarded persons in American society.* Dordrecht, the Netherlands: Kluwer/D. Reidel Publishing Company.
34. Runswick-Cole, K. (2011). Time to end the bias towards inclusive education? *British Journal of Special Education,* 38 (3) 112–120.
35. Department for Education (2011). Support and aspiration: A new approach to special educational needs and disability – a consultation, p. 23. Available at http://media.education.gov.uk/assets/files/pdf/g/green%20paper%20presentation.pdf (retrieved May 2015).
36. Runswick-Cole, 2011. See note 34.
37. Goodley, D. & Runswick-Cole, K. (2011b). The violence of disablism. *Journal of Sociology of Health and Illness,* 33 (4) 602–617, p. 610.
38. Ibid.
39. Runswick-Cole, K. & Hodge, N. (2009). Needs or rights? A challenge to the discourse of special education. *British Journal of Special Education,* 36 (4) 198–203.
40. Goodley & Runswick-Cole, 2011b. See note 37.
41. Ibid. p. 602.
42. Ibid.
43. Ibid. p. 606.
44. Ibid.
45. Ibid.
46. Todd, S. (2002). Death does not become us: The absence of death and dying in intellectual disability research. *Journal of Gerontological Social Work,* 38, 225–239.
47. Milo, E. (1997). Maternal responses to the life and death of a child with a developmental disability: A story of hope. *Death Studies,* 21, 443–476.
48. Ryan, S. (2014). Continuing to get it wrong for learning disabled people and their families: Time to stop 'learning lessons'. Disability Studies Association Conference, University of Lancaster, 9–11 September 2014.
49. Goodley, D. & Runswick-Cole, K. (2010b). Len Barton, inclusion and critical disability studies: Theorising disabled childhoods. *International Studies in Sociology of Education,* 20 (4) 273–290, p. 287.

50. Quoted in Goodley, D. & Runswick-Cole, K. (2012). The body as disability and possibility: Theorising the 'leaking, lacking and excessive' bodies of disabled children. *Scandinavian Journal of Disability Research 15*(1): 1–19.
51. Chesner, A. (1995). *Drama Therapy for People with Learning Difficulties: A world of difference.* London: Jessica Kingsley Publishers.
52. Goodley, D. & Runswick-Cole, K. (2011c). Something in the air? Creativity, culture and community. *Research in Drama Education,* 16 (1) 75.
53. Ibid.
54. Overboe, J. (2004). Articulating a sociology of desire exceeding the normative shadows. Unpublished PhD thesis, Vancouver, University of British Columbia.
55. See http://communitycirclesblog.wordpress.com
56. Haraldsdóttir, F. (2013). Simply Children. In T. Curran & K. Runswick-Cole (Eds). *Disabled Children's Childhood Studies: Critical approaches in a global context* (pp. 13–21). Basingstoke: Palgrave Macmillan.

Chapter 9
Children and electroconvulsive therapy

Craig Newnes

Electrocution is not something to take lightly. I have met numerous individuals electrocuted under the auspices of Psy (and was once hurled across a room by the force of the electric shock consequent on inadvertently jamming a screwdriver into an electric socket). The treatment receives bad press amongst recipients and only occasional press coverage by the media. Phone calls from journalists asking me for quotes about the state of Psy would usually receive the response, 'You're asking the wrong questions. You should be writing about ECT,' with the invariable reply: 'They don't still do that, do they?' But they do, with the complicity of relatives, patients and the press itself, always keen to promote a new 'breakthrough' in treatment for oppression inscribed as depression.

This chapter will look at the history, rationale and research concerning electroconvulsive therapy (ECT) with a group that is in no position to consent and is particularly vulnerable to the effects of being electrocuted – children.

ECT and the Psy complex

There have been campaigns against most Psy treatments for over a century – from the Alleged Lunatics' Friend Society of the mid-nineteenth century to Witness (formerly POPAN) today.[1] There are several websites devoted to critiquing ECT.[2] Facebook and related media are a source of information from ECT survivors.[3] Campaigners aim to make the practice more *visible*.

ECT might be viewed as representative of much that occurs within the Psy complex: the technique has harmed millions; it is based on suspect and ever-changing theoretical assumptions; research is scientistic and carried out exclusively by those with vested interests in the results; it is most commonly used on those with little power who have been marked, frequently via psychometric assessment, in the context of coercion and lack of consent; and – importantly – health professionals are largely silent on the topic. For Erwin Staub, they would be classed as 'bystanders' in the face of harm perpetrated on patients in the same system within which they work.[4]

During ECT an electric current is passed briefly through the brain, via electrodes applied to the scalp, to induce generalised seizure activity. The treatment is usually bilateral (electrodes placed on both temples), though this varies (see below). The person receiving the treatment is anaesthetised; muscle relaxants are given to prevent spasms. This also varies, however, (see below): 'unmodified' ECT – *without* anaesthesia, with consequent skeletal fractures – is practised in Africa, Turkey, Russia, China and some other countries. Melinda James, an ECT survivor, has also questioned the efficacy of the anaesthesia in modified ECT:

> The drug they give to avoid bones breaking is NOT a muscle relaxant. It is a muscle paralyser. It paralyses all the muscles. You cannot blink your eyes, you cannot breathe. I know because one time or maybe more (I only remember one) they did not give me enough of the anaesthetic, and I was not asleep. I could not tell them I was fully conscious – could not move, could not blink my eyes. I saw the doctor leaning over me with the electrodes. Then I was knocked out by the shock. Fully conscious, but paralysed, it felt like someone had bashed my head in with a hammer.[5]

It is recommended that ECT is given twice a week up to a maximum of six weeks; again, this varies (see below). Repeated treatments induce molecular and cellular changes in the brain, characterised by psychiatrist Peter Breggin as 'brain damage' and an 'electrical lobotomy'.[6,7] Weiner agrees, noting that an electroencephalogram (EEG) will detect brain injury following unilateral ECT.[8] Neurologists Symonds and Sament compare the cerebral damage of the practice to head injury.[9,10] Similarly, McClelland sees post-ECT changes as identical to classic signs of frontal lobe damage.[11]

These studies might suggest why ECT continues to be repackaged. A treatment designed to cause brain damage requires a marketing approach that ignores adverse effects while offering a convincing rationale. That rationale is usually absent; the Royal College of Psychiatrists' website is succinct: 'No-one is certain how ECT works.'[12] For the human brain, signs of damage are frequently functional. Few psychiatrists or psychiatric nurses will have seen a patient post-ECT without disturbances in vision, balance or co-ordination.[13] Many will have witnessed in ECT survivors post-treatment memory loss of over six months. The loss of memory is of less concern to clinicians when recipients are elderly; symptoms may be interpreted as features of normal ageing. Thus age as well as the supposed psychiatric disorder can be used to distract relatives, carers and patients from iatrogenic sequaelae.

Assault via electrocution has been foisted on people marked with labels as diverse as schizophrenia and epilepsy. The praxis, popular in services for older people (particularly women), is also promoted for child recipients. One argument presented for this is that children are being 'denied' the right to a treatment with proven efficacy amongst the adult population.[14] ECT is now marketed as a specific treatment for schizophrenia and depression for an age range from four to 104.[15] The next section examines some of the history of electrocuting children.

A history

The ancient Egyptians used electric marine rays to treat epilepsy, and the ancient Romans used the current generated by electric rays for the treatment of headaches, gout, and to assist in obstetrical procedures. The journal *Electricity and Medicine* was first published in 1744. It was claimed here that electric stimuli could be curative for 'neurologic and mental cases of paralysis and epilepsy'.[16] In the 1755 edition, J.B. LeRoy detailed a case of hysterical blindness cured with three applications of electric shock. In 1752 Benjamin Franklin had recorded the use of an 'electro static machine to cure a woman of hysterical fits'.[17] By the mid-nineteenth century Duchenne, the 'father of electrotherapy', was to say, 'No sincere neurologist could practise without the use of electrotherapy.'[18]

By comparison with the catalogue of thousands of somatic treatments, the total of 500 or so present-day psychotherapies attempted with people seen as mad seems positively modest. Trepanning – far from disappearing with the ancient Egyptians – re-emerged with Roger of Salerno in the twelfth century and again in 1899 with Claye Shaw at Banstead Asylum. Rather than freeing spirits, Shaw was attempting to relieve inter-cranial pressure, a presumed cause of general paresis.[19]

The site of inter-cranial pressure was the brain, an organ so little known and so complex that psychiatry has not hesitated to claim jurisdiction over its workings and modification. During the mid-twentieth century neurologists vied with neurosurgeons and psychiatrists for dominance in the field. The first group saw neurosurgeons as useful partners in the enterprise. Psychiatrists were regarded as a profession that should limit themselves to functional disorders of conduct and an ill-defined 'mind'. For psychiatry, however, the brain seemed to show some promise in demonstrating that functional disorders were physically based.[20]

The idiopathic nature of an individual's physical make-up and metabolism, however, renders any medical procedure something of an experiment. ECT is no exception. Effectively, every ECT treatment is an experiment with an N of one. An analogy might be a suggested aeroplane flight where customers are warned that only half of them are likely to arrive at their destination while at least one in a hundred similar flights are known to crash with no survivors. The rhetoric surrounding air travel, and the negative predictions about alternative – possibly already tested – different ways of getting from A to B, will encourage some passengers to take the risk. If that risk is to a relative then the parent, adult, child or sibling may agree that the person inscribed as depressed or psychotic should take the flight. The next section discusses ECT in relation to praxis with children, where a parent is frequently the person giving consent.

ECT with children

Child and adolescent mental health services are ambiguous concerning their definition of childhood (see Chapter 1). As noted there, in the UK NHS, different regions and health administrative structures differ in their definitions of the points at which a child becomes an adolescent and then an adult. For some the definitions depend on education: a child becomes an adolescent when she enters secondary education, becoming an adult when she leaves the school system. For others there are age demarcations: 'children' remain children until age 13 and are adolescents until, roughly, 20; adolescents are teenagers. For others 'children' effectively become 'adults' if child services cannot cope – many patients have been admitted, aged 10, to psychiatric hospitals since the nineteenth century.[21] Beyond the confines of structuralised service definitions, for many parents their children remain 'children' all their lives. Mothers may still refer to sons as 'boys' or daughters as 'girls' long past the point they have reached adulthood. For parents whose offspring never leave home or, due to being marked as 'disabled', have been institutionalised, the social context re-languages the child as 'lazy', 'dependent', or, in the case of those with physical disabilities or psychiatric diagnoses, 'eternally innocent' or 'tragic'. Service definitions of childhood reflect wider societal ambiguities: in the UK a 10-year-old can be tried for murder, but that same child would have to wait until 16 to legally begin a consensual sexual relationship, 17 to drive, 18 to vote, etc. In the USA, the age demarcation lines differ between states for driving, owning a gun and buying alcohol.

The brain, however, continues to develop throughout adolescence. For neurologists it is undisputed that the developing brain is vulnerable; any assault on brain tissue – whether it be biochemical, traumatic or through ECT – is injurious to brain cells and neuronal connections.

In 1947 child neuropsychiatrist Lauretta Bender (to become famous as the progenitor of the Bender-Gestalt test) published a study carried out on 98 children aged between four and 11 years old who had been treated in the previous five years with intensive courses of electroconvulsive therapy (ECT). Most were inscribed with 'childhood schizophrenia'. These children received ECT daily for a typical course of approximately 20 treatments,[22] an intensive regime first suggested by Bini and known as regressive ECT or annihilation therapy.[23] Beneficial effects of ECT were reported in the majority but complete remission was rare. Bender abandoned the use of ECT in the 1950s. Her published work on the use of ECT in children was discredited after a study showing that the children had either not improved or had been harmed.[24]

During the 1960s Bender supervised the children's unit of Creedmoor Hospital. It has been described as a 'veritable snake pit'.[25] Her assessment technique consisted of an interview with the child, followed by analysis of the child's responses and conduct in front of a large group of staff and the child, as though the latter could not hear. The technique bears comparison with the earlier work of Gesell (see Chapter 1): work that made the child the object of study and inscription as if the researchers were irrelevant. Bender performed a 'diagnostic test' on children, which involved holding the head of a standing child and gently turning it. Supposedly, schizophrenic children would turn in the direction of the pressure and normal children would resist.[26] Comparison may be made with any number of scientific and unsophisticated procedures within Psy from the 'blank-screen' of classical psychoanalysis, via Eysenck's reaction time experiments using *string* to measure so-called introversion, to the production of norms for assessment tools such as the Stroop Test. For the latter, much of the experimental development uses psychology undergraduates rewarded with course credits for their participation.

Research on ECT with children

Research in Psy is bedevilled by methodological and philosophical questions. Psy diagnostic schemata are both unreliable and invalid, and depend on notions of interiority and individuality that are impossible to verify by the methods of science. The *questions* posed within Psy research mimic the hypotheses of science while research subjects, humans, are in a *relationship* with researchers that is transitory and non-replicable. A combination of the publishing imperative (for academic researchers), the promise of cultural (and financial) capital, curiosity and a deeply ironic lack of reflexivity maintains research praxis in the face of nosological, methodological or philosophical challenges. Research is what researchers *do*.

Research concerning ECT with children is, possibly, more suspect than other research in Psy, as outlined below.

Rey and Walter discuss an example of a 15-year-old girl diagnosed with schizophrenia who received 200 ECT treatments in one year. More dramatically, a 16-year-old girl diagnosed as suffering from dementia praecox was treated with 15 unmodified ECTs in three days. She developed an organic brain syndrome over a period of three weeks. Five other patients were reported to have ended the ECT prematurely due to adverse effects. These included a depressed teenager who was considered 'manic' after five ECTs, two whose treatment was discontinued because of increasing agitation, one who showed marked confusion after two treatments and an 18-year-old woman diagnosed with bipolar disorder who developed neuroleptic malignant syndrome following *one* ECT.[27]

Writing in *Convulsive Therapy*, Cohen and colleagues reviewed the medical records of 21 children aged between 13 and 19 who had received bilateral ECT from 1984 to 1995. They found a 40 per cent relapse rate after a year. Partial 'clinical improvement' occurred for some 'schizophrenic and schizoaffective episodes'. Adverse effects were transient but 'frequent'. The researchers concluded that 'ECT is a safe and effective treatment for adolescents with severe and intractable mental illness.'[28] As half of the recipients relapsed and adverse effects were acknowledged as frequent, this seems a conservative reading of the data.

The conclusion exactly mimics promotional literature from both the American Psychiatric Association and Britain's Royal College of Psychiatrists. The latter body has published the definitive guide to ECT. After 300 pages reviewing the evidence to date detailing adverse effects from memory loss (in a third of recipients) to death (frequently as a result of the anaesthetic rather than the electric shocks) the Royal College *Handbook* ends with a few pages on what to tell prospective patients and relatives. The first recommendation is that people be informed the treatment is, indeed, 'safe and effective'.[29]

Numerous studies and reviews come to a similar conclusion. Wachtel and colleagues suggest that 'the indications for electroconvulsive therapy in children and adolescents are similar to those in adults, including severe affective, psychotic and catatonic pathology'. Arguing that it is bad publicity that prevents clinicians and parents considering ECT as an option, they urge the 'removal of impediments to ECT access in this population', adding that children diagnosed with autism and neurodevelopmental disabilities should also be candidates.[30] A further study examines ECT treatment of a 14-year-old boy marked with moderate learning disability and autism. His existing catatonic stupor required him to have nasogastric nutrition and fluid replacement. Antidepressant treatment had not helped and zolpidem produced only a temporary improvement in the catatonia. The authors conclude that bilateral ECT 'produced a significant response after the third treatment, and progressive improvement to the end of the course of 13 sessions'. In a classic example of reverse logic the authors suggest: 'Successful maintenance on a neuroleptic–lithium combination and previous episodes of catatonic excitement are suggestive of an underlying bipolar disorder.'[31] This is not unlike concluding that because a plaster cast helped a person walk better she must have had a broken leg when closer examination would have revealed that her legs were tied together.

In Israel a study compared the results of ECT in two groups (adolescents and adults) in a community psychiatric institution. The files of 24 consecutive adolescent patients treated in the years 1991 to 1995 were retrospectively examined, and the findings were compared with those in 33 adult patients who started their ECT course on the same day. The authors conclude that ECT was equally effective for adolescents and adults (58 per cent in each group achieved remission).[32]

Willoughby reports a case study of *one* 8-year-old girl diagnosed with psychotic depression and concludes, 'Nurses and other healthcare personnel should consider ECT in refractory cases of major depressive disorder, bipolar affective disorder, schizophrenia, and other psychotic disorders.'[33]

In July 2002 the Brazilian Federal Council of Medicine, in its Resolution n. 1640, regulated the use of electroconvulsive therapy in Brazil. It prohibited the use of ECT in patients below 16 years of age, unless in exceptional circumstances.[34] Partly in response to this resolution, Lima and colleagues conducted an extensive review of ECT use with young people. Lima and colleagues define adolescence as the 'state of being 13 to 18 years of age' and surveyed three medical databases: PMC (United States National Library of Medicine), LILACS (Literatura Latino-Americana e do Caribe em Ciências da Saúde), and SciELO (Scientific Electronic Library Online).

The research is something of an object lesson in the academy's demand for publication; there are 16 authors named in a study that was, in effect, a literature search and review.

Inclusion criteria were: (1) manuscripts written in English, Portuguese, Spanish or French; (2) case reports, series of cases, case-controls, literature reviews, cross-sectional studies, exploratory field research, and prospective and retrospective cohort studies; (3) studies regarding the use of ECT in adolescents, provided they respected at least three of the five PICOS criteria: adolescent, ECT, absent or only drugs, symptoms remission, and study design. Studies assessing other conditions, editorials and letters to the editor were excluded. From the 212 studies surveyed the authors reduced their final total to 33, a further six being added from research referenced in the reviewed sample.[35]

The authors conclude that ECT use in adolescents is 'considered a highly efficient option for treating several psychiatric disorders, achieving high remission rates, and presenting few and relatively benign adverse effects'.[36] In their introduction they suggest that adolescents experience 'self-destruction impulses'. (The authors do not reflect on the possibility that agreeing to ECT is, in itself, self-destructive.) They go on to describe the introduction of ECT as a revolution in psychiatry. This rhetorical device sets the scene for what follows. The authors are not able to make a morally grounded statement concerning ECT use, partly because their approach is not neutral and partly because morally based reasoning cannot be applied to these kinds of data; studies of this type always reveal a mixture of success and failure in the preferred treatment strategy. The *only* criterion used by researchers in recommending continuation of the treatment under review is an implicit appeal to Bentham's notion of 'the greater good'. If, for example, two children die and 20 others have profound cognitive deficits in a sample of 100 children given ECT, authors will conclude that those deaths and adverse effects are compensated for by the 40 children who showed no relapse after a year. The benefits are seen to outweigh the risks. This, however, is only one way to judge 'benefit' and deliberately ignores the Hippocratic Oath's requirement to 'first do no harm'. A consent form beginning with the words 'I understand I may die but my death may benefit others in the future' would be a challenging addition to the existing pre-treatment literature. At present, consent forms are limited to acknowledging headache, nausea and vomiting, agitation, and mental confusion as the most common adverse effects.[37]

The authors note that the American Academy of Child and Adolescent Psychiatry (AACAP) has established that eligibility for ECT in adolescents involves meeting three criteria: (1) diagnosis, (2) severity of symptoms, (3) lack of treatment response to appropriate psychopharmacological agents accompanied by other appropriate treatment modalities. ECT is recommended for adolescents with diagnoses such as persistent major depression, schizoaffective disorder, schizophrenia, or history of manic episodes, with or without psychotic features.[38] Other researchers have suggested that ECT can be used with child and adolescent populations to treat catatonia and neuroleptic malignant syndrome.[39,40] The latter is one adverse effect of neuroleptic medication. Here *further* brain damage is being recommended as a treatment for iatrogenic harm.

Notwithstanding the lack of validity in Psy diagnoses, ECT is most frequently used with children labelled depressed – a supposed 'mood disorder'. It has also been used with children and adolescents inscribed as 'bipolar', 'mentally retarded', 'autistic', 'schizophrenic', and 'endogenously depressed'.[41,42,43,44,45] This last illustrates the unreliability of using even relatively recent research to support contemporary treatments in the field; 'endogenous' depression was removed from the official lexicon over 30 years ago.

Three studies retrieved by Lima et al. compared ECT use in adolescents with ECT use in patients of other ages. Adolescents subjected to ECT account for only 0.43 per cent of the total treatments in India, 0.93 per cent in Australia and 1.5 per cent in the USA.[46,47,48] A study from New South Wales involves a 53-item telephone survey with people who received ECT before the age of 19 years. Opinions about ECT were generally positive; the majority considered ECT a legitimate treatment and would have ECT again and recommend it to others.[49]

Medicare figures show the use of ECT has tripled in Victoria state in Australia in the private health sector in six years. In 2007–2008, 18,000 treatments were conducted. In Victoria's private health system ECT use increased from 1,944 treatments in 2001–2002 to 6,009 in 2007–2008. Of the 18,000 reported treatments, 12,000 were in the public health system. Of these 18,000, 6,197 ECT treatments were compulsory and nearly three times as many women had shock treatment compared with men. Increasing numbers of patients who had been forced into ECT treatment contacted the Mental Health Legal Centre claiming they were tortured. Throughout Australia there were 203 ECT treatments on children younger than 14 – including 55 carried out on children aged four and younger. Two of the under-fours were in Victoria.[50]

Finally, Lima and colleagues conclude: 'ECT is the treatment of choice depending on diagnosis, severity of symptoms, and lack of response to psychopharmacotherapy. The majority of the studies in the scientific literature show the efficiency of ECT use in adolescents and consider this approach more efficient than psychopharmacotherapy isolated [sic].' And, 'an experienced staff and adequate physical conditions can minimize the risk of complications'. Iatrogenic harm is thus reduced to 'complications'.[51]

In contrast, Jones and Baldwin remark, 'ECT has been repackaged in a manner designed to censor public opinion. Empirical research, based on adequate methodological data, does not exist.'[52]

The lack of controlled studies is a common concern amongst ECT reviewers. A recent review of ECT with children marked as learning disabled found no controlled studies, the majority of articles consisting of case reports. The authors performed an online literature search for national and international journal articles published before March 2010. They found 72 case reports, a retrospective chart review study and other reviews, but no controlled studies. Despite the lack of rigour the review suggests that 'Most patients (79%) showed a positive outcome following ECT. Complications were seen only in 13 per cent and there were no reports of cognitive decline.' Many patients, however, relapsed following ECT (32%), the majority being medicated at follow-up (71%).[53]

Despite these results and concerns that 'the sample is relatively small and there is a definite skew in the severity of intellectual disability represented, with the majority of case reports being of patients with mild and moderate disability,' the authors conclude: 'Electroconvulsive therapy is a valuable treatment for this patient group and should be considered earlier as opposed to as a last resort.' The identified obstacles to its use noted by the authors include 'diagnostic difficulties, ethical and legal issues, a lack of objective measurements and uncertainty about its safety in this population'.[54]

Other authors see few ethical challenges: 'If patients with intellectual disability are likely to suffer more because of ... medications and their inability to report somatic side-effects, it may be that ECT would benefit them by reducing the need for multiple medications.'[55] This reasoning has led others to conclude: 'In specific patients [children inscribed as learning disabled], ECT may actually be the more conservative treatment option.'[56]

Worldwide, ECT is used in different ways with different populations, an inconsistency to be found in all Psy treatments across and within countries. In Spain in the 1990s 17 per cent of ECT patients were being treated for schizophrenia; the figure was similar for France. In Texas (one of the few states in the US for which information on ECT use is available) in the same decade just under 10 per cent of ECT patients had a diagnosis of schizophrenia or schizoaffective disorder, while in Kuwait an inscription of schizophrenia was the most common indication for ECT, accounting for nearly 40 per cent of patients. In Hungary in 2002 over half of ECT patients had a diagnosis of schizophrenia, and in Australia in the early 2000s nearly 10 per cent of ECT patients had a diagnosis of schizophrenia. Over the same period in Asia schizophrenia was the most common diagnosis for ECT patients, accounting for over 40 per cent of medicalised assaults.[57]

For some, the dividing line between treatment and torture is difficult to discern. Following a two-year investigation, Mental Disability Rights International (MDRI) released a report detailing the human rights abuses perpetrated in Turkey against children and adults in the Psy system. *Behind Closed Doors: Human rights abuses in the psychiatric facilities, orphanages and rehabilitation centers of Turkey* describes the widespread use of ECT on psychiatric patients as young as nine years old without the use of anaesthesia. The investigators also found evidence of children dying from starvation, dehydration and lack of medical care in 'residential rehabilitation centres'. The report documents Turkey's violations of the European Convention for the Prevention of Torture (ECPT), the European Convention on Human Rights (ECHR), the UN Convention on the Rights of the Child (CRC) and other internationally accepted human rights and disability rights standards.[58]

Herman and colleagues showed that rates of ECT use across US states were highly variable, higher than for most medical and surgical procedures. In some urban areas, access to ECT is limited. In 13 US states ECT is regulated by law, and in Colorado and Texas it is forbidden for children under 16. In Missouri a court order is needed. In Tennessee a child can be electroshocked only for 'mania or severe depression'.[59] For some ECT proponents this is a denial of the 'right' to be electrocuted at a psychiatrist's behest. Shorter objects to such regulation and claims ECT is the 'penicillin of psychiatry'. He states, 'The legislative overreach concerning ECT in children leaves one open-mouthed … This is ageism in reverse, and terribly unfair,' and asks, 'Are we denying children access to a treatment that is safe and effective in adults?'[60] Shorter uses a rhetorical move, saying that Scientologists (vilified and depicted as a deranged cult in mass media), under the guise of various front organisations, lobby for tightening the ECT restrictions rather than loosening them. The implication is that any right-thinking American would support something Scientology wishes to ban.

The poor public image of the procedure and 'safe and effective' rhetoric is further addressed in a web-based article titled, 'ECT in kids: Safe, effective, robust and… underutilized'.[61] The article reports on a 20-year retrospective study by investigators at the Mayo Clinic in Rochester, Minnesota, presented at the American Psychiatric Association's 2013 Annual Meeting.[62] The Mayo is one of the few centres in the United States using ECT with children and adolescents. The presenters claimed that the procedure reduced 'symptoms of affective disorders, psychotic disorders, and other disorders' up to one year post-treatment with a single series of ECT. They noted that a poor public image and the controversy over its use have led to subsequent underutilisation of ECT and suggested that the image was based on 'outdated misconceptions'.[63]

At the Mayo Clinic, ECT is carried out under the supervision of an anaesthesiologist as well as a psychiatrist. For the study, the investigators examined the medical records of all patients from the ages of 12 to 19 years treated with ECT at the Mayo Clinic from 1993 to 2012. The study included 46 patients; one-year follow-up data were available for 29 of the patients.

The majority were marked as 'suffering from severe, recalcitrant, and frequently comorbid mood, anxiety, and psychotic illnesses — with about an even split between recurrent major depressive disorder and primary psychotic disorder. Other disorders included anorexia nervosa, catatonia, and schizoaffective disorder'. Most were on at least four psychoactive medications simultaneously; the researchers make no causal link between the effects of these medications and the various 'disorders'. The most common adverse effects of ECT were nausea (15.2%) and headaches (13%), followed by 'post-emergent agitation' (8.7%) and spontaneous seizure (4.3%). The presenters concluded that 'ECT remains the gold standard for severe illness.'[64]

Selling shock treatment

Research articles and reviews of ECT are almost comedic in their repetition of the terms 'safe' and 'effective'. A cynic might be tempted to ask why researchers need to repeat these key words so often. Perhaps researchers are trying to convince themselves that electrocuting a child is a perfectly normal thing to do. The repetition echoes the warning given to the character played by Cameron Diaz in *Knight and Day*: 'If someone says to trust him and you are going to be safe, run, they are probably going to kill you.'[65]

The promotional campaign for ECT is not limited to the public. A paper in *Electroconvulsive Therapy* examined the knowledge, experience and attitudes towards the use of electroconvulsive treatment in minors among child and adolescent psychiatrists and psychologists. A majority of the respondents said they had minimal knowledge about the use of ECT in children and adolescents. Lack of confidence in providing a second opinion was reported by three-quarters of respondents. The majority regarded ECT as a treatment of last resort. Compared with those with minimal knowledge, respondents with 'advanced knowledge' reported a higher perception of safety and efficacy, perhaps unsurprising given the constant repetition of the 'safe and effective' claim.[66]

A review of placebo-controlled studies that compared 'sham' ECT with real ECT for depression found that 'real ECT is no more effective than placebo, except during the period of time the ECT is being administered [and] even that difference is modest'. It concludes that 'the effectiveness of ECT is over-endorsed repeatedly in the psychiatric literature'.[67] The Canadian Psychiatric Association (CPA) prefers to state, 'Although a *safe and effective* treatment, ECT remains controversial,' (my italics) and continues, 'In placebo ECT, the patient has exactly the same things done to them – including going to the ECT rooms and having the anaesthetic and muscle relaxant – but no electrical current is passed and there is no fit. In these studies, the patients who had standard ECT were much more likely to recover, and did so more quickly than those who had the placebo treatment.'[68] This position contrasts with the widely held view that – whatever the damaging effects to the brain of electrocution – the mortality rate in ECT is due to anaesthesia. Finally, the CPA underlines efficacy and safety: 'When used properly, ECT is a *safe and effective* treatment which should continue to be available as a therapeutic option for the treatment of mental disorders' (my emphasis).[69]

Publishers too must have some confidence in these promotional exercises by ECT proponents. In 2013 Oxford University Press published *Electroconvulsive Therapy in Children and Adolescents*.[70]

Two (essentially pro-ECT) studies have detailed the necessary *medical* procedures necessary when considering electroshock. The first looked at adults referred for ECT and found that they have a greater number of pathological lesions of the central nervous system identified by a CT or MRI scan. The author suggests that some of these lesions may affect treatment outcome or seizure duration. Therefore, an MRI or CT scan is indicated in adolescents *before* ECT, a costly recommendation unlikely to be carried out even by those few who have read the study.[71] The second study examined the effectiveness and safety of ECT in 'pharmacotherapy-refractory depression' in 11 hospitalised adolescents. A potentially serious complication of tardive seizure occurred in one recipient. Prolonged seizures were noted in seven of the 11 patients. Pending further research on ECT in youth, the authors recommended that ECT should only be administered to youth in hospital settings, that *all* regularly administered psychotropic medications (including antidepressants) be discontinued before ECT, and that physicians be aware that 12 treatments are 'usually sufficient'.[72] It is unknown how many ECT practitioners follow these recommendations. The recommendations, however, remain part of rhetoric consistent with the notion that professionals should be trusted – and *may* be held to account if not following guidelines claimed to enhance 'safety'.

From controversy to illegality

The repackaging and marketing of ECT continues. ECT is predominantly confined to older women and performed with the consent of relatives or with the approval, in the UK, of Second Opinion Doctors. Any 'controversy' is limited by the lack of publicity for the praxis and its invisibility within the clinic. For children and adolescents any debate is mostly confined to anti-ECT activists (frequently online) and within the pages of psychiatric journals. Acknowledgement that social factors are a major (some might suggest sole) determinant of the likelihood of being marked as depressed does not lead Psy practitioners to suggest social intervention.

The appeal to notions of interiority and individuality is exemplified in the 'American Indian and Alaska Native Women and Depression FACT SHEET', available on the National Alliance on Mental Illness website – 'Many minority women experience depression and stress brought on by persistent racism, gender bias, violence, poverty, large family size and social disadvantages.' Suggested amelioration of the misery brought on by such circumstances involves only the *nonsequitur* of Psy intervention: 'medications, psychotherapy and electroconvulsive therapy (ECT). For people who have a seasonal component to their depression, light therapy may be useful.'[73] This can be read as a further colonialising move; as in any colonised culture the language and mores of the invading culture soon overwhelm the existing customs. The – for some – romanticised view of indigenous culture is one of spirituality and community. Disruption to that spirituality and sense of cohesion is met, by the invading culture, with further oppression in the form of technical Psy praxis. Thus, for indigenous (First People) Australians and Native Americans, rates of mental illness diagnoses and subsequent treatments such as ECT are in excess of the rates for other citizens.[74]

As ECT is more frequently given to older people there are more women in the target group. Other tentative hypotheses might include a more general antagonism to women from the male-dominated Psy complex.[75] More radically, it is possible that '"depression" is identified in a group who are actually exhausted by their multiple societal roles and who have less support for their travails'.[76]

Research criteria invariably involve the subjects under scrutiny. Criteria for *researchers* rarely go beyond a brief allusion to their academic qualifications. Research on ECT (a treatment designed to destroy brain cells, neuronal connections and memory) should, perhaps, include criteria for those very researchers. Do we know, for example, if the researchers are parents? If they are, do we know if they *like* children? The scientific ethos in Psy presumes that researchers are neutral observers. It is clear, however, that some people do not like children. Any parent is likely to go through periods of wanting offspring to leave home as soon as possible. Adults who are not parents may regard their lack of offspring as a choice, based on not particularly liking or valuing children.

For children and teenagers there is no guarantee of sympathy from adults and adult researchers. One criterion for researchers might then be to answer, as honestly as possible, '*Why* do you think you want to electrocute young people?' The vested interest would be in profiting through the satisfaction of harming people rather than material gain (the interest declared as a 'conflict of interest' in journal articles). Science demands the most parsimonious theories to explain results. Uncomfortable though it certainly is to contemplate the possibility that Psy professionals set out to harm patients, particularly children, this is one hypothesis that might bear further scrutiny.

A further hypothesised motivation is that psychiatrists continue to promote physical interventions in order to place the discipline within the bounds of 'real' medicine: that is, medicine that deals with physically verifiable illness in physical ways. This position is made clear in an editorial from the *American Journal of Psychiatry*:

> Since the mind is the organ expression of the activity of the brain, we can hope that some day we will achieve a complete understanding of all mental illnesses as both mind and brain diseases. And that psychiatry will still exist until the illnesses themselves cease to exist – as the medical specialty responsible for the study and treatment of mental illnesses.[77]

Some activists, unimpressed by the psychiatric drive for acceptance as *bona fide* medical doctors, have pressed for changes in the law. For adults ECT is illegal only in Slovenia. To date the only country to have ratified the use of advance directives is Germany.[78] To that extent psychiatric patients are only safe from electroshock in Slovenia (where psychiatrists continue to refer potential recipients over the border to Croatia) or, as German citizens, if they have signed an advance directive stating they do not want to receive electroshock in Germany. Children, however, as minors, are not protected by the law. Mental health legislation in Western Australia banning the use of ECT on those under 14 passed through State Parliament in October 2014. The law imposes a $15,000 fine on anyone performing the therapy on a child under 14. A child aged between 14 and 18 who is a voluntary patient cannot have the treatment without informed consent and approval by the Mental Health Tribunal.[79]

For many Psy professionals, use of ECT with children is condoned only *in extremis* and where it might be described as 'life saving'. As noted above, some psychiatrists recommend ECT as the preferred choice of intervention, an argument made on its behalf for older people and in pregnant women. Aziz and colleagues suggest that ECT should be seen as 'the more conservative option' for people marked as autistic.[80] I have described elsewhere how the criteria for a diagnosis of autism has expanded to involve a 'spectrum' wherein almost any child can lie on the spectrum, as it incorporates many behaviours, however undesirable, that are common amongst children.[81] If ECT is seen as a first treatment for those marked as autistic, then an informed consent form as follows may be the way forward for concerned parents and carers:

> Your child has received a psychiatric diagnosis. This label has no validity but may be based on a foreign language so it sounds impressive. Your consultant may or may not like children and has a history of electrocuting them. The electric shocks will destroy brain cells and will have little effect

in the long term on the behaviour of your child, who will continue to be medicated with a variety of harmful drugs. There is a small chance of your child dying from the electric shock or anaesthesia.

Magic and the future of ECT

Magic has long been a component of Psy theorising and praxis. This magic is contextual and shifts within a wider zeitgeist. Thus counselling, mindfulness, psychopharmacology and other Psy interventions rely on mysterious processes and biochemical changes both invisible and unknown (despite many competing hypotheses) to patients and professionals. Appeals to broad constructs such as 'connectedness', 'community', or 'mind' continue alongside more specific notions of 'brain-biochemical imbalance' or 'genetic predisposition'. All such constructs are, by necessity, metaphorical. The language of Psy borrows from and lends to a wider discourse of individuality and interiority where 'selves' are constructed and behaviour inscribed in Psy terminology by the public as much as by Psy experts. The magic inherent in this discourse involves, in the case of ECT, a further appeal to the culturally valued tropes of 'science' and 'research'.

It is this cultural value, rather than any proven benefit to patients, that will maintain the use of ECT with children. As experts and the public are less beguiled by the mysteries of electricity, the praxis will, like insulin-coma therapy and trans-orbital lobotomy before it, become a historical footnote in the annals of Psy, of value to publishers and historians who will, perhaps, shock us metaphorically rather than literally.

Dedication

This chapter is dedicated to the memory of Professor Steve Baldwin and Leonard Roy Frank.

Endnotes

1. http://www.wherecanifind.net/cgi-bin/callentry.cgi?255 (retrieved 15 March 2015).
2. See, for example, http://intcamp.wordpress.com/ban-ect/ and http://camhjournal.com/2012/04/24/2004-a-campaign-against-direct-ect/
3. See, for example, ECT Global Support https://www.facebook.com/groups/414257808688052/ and Mind Freedom Ireland http://www.mindfreedomireland.com/
4. Staub, E. (1989). *The Roots of Evil: The origins of genocide and other group violence.*

New York: Cambridge University Press. For examples of clinical psychologists speaking out via publication, see Baldwin, S. & Jones, Y. (1990). ECT, children and clinical psychologists: A shock to the system? *Clinical Psychology Forum, 25,* 2–4; Johnstone, L. (1999). Adverse psychological effects of ECT. *Journal of Mental Health,* 8 (1) 69–85; Johnstone, L. (2002). *Users and Abusers of Psychiatry: A critical look at psychiatric practice* (2nd ed.). London: Routledge.

5. James, M. Available at http://ectstatistics.wordpress.com/2013/05/20/75- years-of-electroconvulsive-therapy/ (retrieved 30 May 2013).

6. Breggin, P. (1991). *Toxic Psychiatry: Why therapy, empathy and love must replace the drugs, electroshock, and biochemical theories of the 'new psychiatry'.* New York: St. Martin's Press.

7. Breggin, P. R. (1998). Electroshock: Scientific, ethical, and political issues. *International Journal of Risk & Safety in Medicine, 11,* 5–40.

8. Weiner, R. D. (1980). The persistence of ECT-induced changes in the electro encephalogram. *Journal of Mental Disease, 168,* 224–228.

9. Symonds, C. P. (1966). Disorders of memory. *Brain, 89,* 625–640.

10. S. Sament quoted in Frank, L. R. (1990). Electroshock: Death, brain damage, memory loss and brainwashing. *Journal of Mind and Behaviour, II* (3–4) 489–512.

11. McClelland, R. J. (1988). Psychosocial sequelae of head injury: An anatomy of a relationship. *British Journal of Psychaitry, 153,* 141–146.

12. Royal College of Psychiatrists. Information on ECT. Available at http://www.rcpsych.ac.uk/healthadvice/treatmentswellbeing.aspx#E (retrieved 16 March 2015).

13. For a patient-centred account of the immediate effects of ECT (the camera angle positions the viewer as the recipient of the treatment) see *We're Not Mad, We're Angry,* a Channel 4 'Eleventh Hour' documentary made in 1986. Available at www.youtube.com/watch?v=qD36m1mveoY (retrieved, 17 March 2015).

14. Shorter, E. (2013). Electroconvulsive therapy in children. *How Everyone Became Depressed.* Available at http://www.psychologytoday.com/blog/how-everyone-became-depressed/201312/electroconvulsive-therapy-in-children (retrieved 4 August 2014).

15. Jones, Y. & Baldwin, S. (1992). ECT: Shock, lies and psychiatry. *Changes: An International Journal of Psychology and Psychotherapy, 10* (2) 126–135.

16. Harm, E. (1955). The origin and early history of electrotherapy and electroshock. *American Journal of Psychiatry, 111,* 933.

17. Quoted in Palmer, R. L. (1981). The history of shock treatment. In R. L. Palmer (Ed.). *Electroconvulsive Therapy: An appraisal.* Oxford: Oxford University Press, p. 3.

18. Quoted in Harm, 1955. See note 16.

19. Stone, M. (1998). *Healing the Mind: A history of psychiatry from antiquity to the present.* London: Pimlico, p. 8.

20. Attempts to link madness to genuine organic pathology (other than that caused by medication) continue. A study from Chicago's Northwestern University screened the blood of teenagers for 26 markers found to be present in those with depression (according to animal studies). Britain's *Daily Telegraph,* explicitly reports, 'Finding a biological sign of depression also confirms that the condition is a disease.' (Smith, R. (2014). Chemical link to teenagers with depression. *The Daily Telegraph,* September 15, p. 13.)

21. Newnes, C. (2015). Chapter 3. In *Inscription, Diagnosis and Deception in the Mental Health Industry: How Psy governs us all.* Basingstoke: Palgrave Macmillan.

22. Bender, L. (1947). One hundred cases of childhood schizophrenia treated with electric shock. *Transactions of the American Neurological Society, 72,* 165–169. Quoted in Rey, J. M. & Walter, G. (1997). Half a century of ECT use in young people. *American Journal of Psychiatry, 154,* (5) 595–602, p. 596.

23. Shorter, E. & Healy, D. (2007). *Shock Therapy: A history of electroconvulsive treatment in mental illness*. New Brunswick, NJ: Rutgers University Press, p. 137.
24. Boodman, S. G. (1996). Shock therapy: It's back. *Washington Post*, 24 September, 14–20.
25. Decker, H. (2013). *The Making of DSM-IIIRG: A Diagnostic Manual's conquest of American psychiatry*. Oxford: Oxford University Press.
26. Wikipedia (n.d.). Lauretta Bender. Available at http://www.en.wikipedia.org/wiki/Lauretta_Bender (retrieved 9 March 2015).
27. Rey, J. M. & Walter, G. (1997). Half a century of ECT use in young people. *American Journal of Psychiatry, 154* (5) 595–602.
28. Cohen, D., Paillère-Martinot, M. L. & Basquin, M. (1997). Use of electroconvulsive therapy in adolescents. *Convulsive Therapy, 13* (1) 25–31.
29. Arscott, K. (1999). ECT: The facts psychiatry declines to mention. In C. Newnes, G. Holmes & C. Dunn (Eds). *This is Madness: A critical look at psychiatry and the future of mental health services* (pp. 97–118). Ross-on-Wye: PCCS Books.
30. Wachtel, L. E., Dhossche, D. M. & Kellner, C. H. (2011). When is electroconvulsive therapy appropriate for children and adolescents? *Medical Hypotheses, 76* (3) 395–399.
31. Zaw, F. K. M., Bates, G. D. L., Murali, V., et al. (1999). Catatonia, autism and ECT. *Developmental Medicine and Child Neurology, 41*, 843–845. Quoted in Muir, P. J. (2005). The use of ECT in people with learning disability. In A. I. F. Scott (Ed.). *The ECT Handbook, Second Edition: The third report of the Royal College of Psychiatrists' Special Committee on ECT* (pp. 57–67). Gaskell: RCP, p. 62.
32. Bloch, Y., Levcovitch, Y., Bloch, A. M. & Mendlovic, S. (2001). Electroconvulsive therapy in adolescents: Similarities to and differences from adults. *Journal of the American Academy of Child and Adolescent Psychiatry, 40* (11) 1332–1336.
33. Willoughby, C. L., Hradek, E. A. & Richards, N. R. (1997). Use of electroconvulsive therapy with children: An overview and case report. *Journal of Child and Adolescent Psychiatric Nursing, 10* (3) 11–17.
34. Conselho Federal de Medicina (Brazilian Federal Council of Medicine) (2002). *Resolução CFM N° 1640/2002. Dispõe sobre a eletroconvulsoterapia e dá outras providências* [PubMed Abstract]. Brasília: CFM.
35. Lima, N. N. R., Nascimento, V. B., Peixoto, J. A. C., Moreira, M. M., Neto, M. L. R., Almeida, J. C., Vasconcelos, C.A.C., Teixeira, S. A., Júnior, J. G., Junior, F.T.C., Guimarães, D.D.M., Brasil, A. Q., Cartaxo, J. S., Akerman, M. & Reis, A.O.A. (2013). Electroconvulsive therapy use in adolescents: A systematic review. *Annals of General Psychiatry 12* (17). Available at http://www.annals-general-psychiatry.com/content/12/1/17 (retrieved 1 May 2015). Lima et al. use the PRISMA protocol for their analysis. See Moher, D., Liberati, A., Tetzlaff, I. & Altman, D. G. (2009). Preferred reporting items for systematic reviews and meta-analyses: The PRISMA statement. *PLoS Med, 6* (7) e10097.
36. *Ibid*.
37. Feliu, M., Edwards, C. L., Sudhakar, S., McDougald, C., Raynor, R. & Johnson, S. (2008). Neuropsychological effects and attitudes in patients following electroconvulsive therapy. *Neuropsychiatric Disease Treatment 4* (3) 613–617.
38. AACAP Official Action (2004). Practice parameter for use of electroconvulsive therapy with adolescents. *Journal of the American Academy of Child and Adolescent Psychiatry, 43*, (12) 1521–1539. The authors claim that 'mood disorders' have a high rate of response to ECT (75–100%); 'psychotic disorders' have a lower response rate (50–60%). See also Salleh, M. A., Papakostas, I., Zervas, I. & Christodoulou, G. (2006). Eletroconvulsoterapia: Critérios e recomendações da Associação Mundial de Psiquiatria. *Review Psiquiatrica Clinicale, 33* (5) 262–267.
39. Consoli, A., Benmiloud, M., Wachtel, L., Dhossche, D., Cohen, D. & Bonnot, O. (2010). Electroconvulsive therapy in adolescents with the catatonia syndrome: Efficacy and ethics. *Journal of Electroconvulsive Therapy, 26* (4) 259–265.

40. Daly, J. J., Prudic, J., Devanand, D. P., Nobler, M. S., Lisanby, S. H., Peyser, S., Roose, S. P. & Sackheim, H. A. (2001). ECT in bipolar and unipolar depression: Differences in speed of response. *Bipolar Disorder 3* (2) 95–104.
41. Kutcher, S. & Robertson, H. A. (1995). Electroconvulsive therapy in treatment resistant bipolar youth. *Journal of Child and Adolescent Psychopharmacology, 5,* 167–175. The authors suggest that ECT *might* be an effective and cost-effective treatment in adolescents with bipolar disorder, in acute mania or a depressive state. In 2014 Soreff and colleagues suggested the 'usefulness' of ECT with patients marked as 'bi-polar'. In 1988 Soreff had been banned from practising medicine in Maine due to sexual relationships with three female patients. He now works in Boston, MA (Soreff., S, McInnes, L. & Ahmed, I. (2014). Bipolar Affective Disorder. Available at emedicine.medscape.com/article/286342-overview (retrieved 5 August 2014).
42. van Waarde, J. A., Stolker, J. J. & van der Mast, R. C. (2001). ECT in mental retardation: A review. *Journal of Electroconvulsive Therapy, 17* (4) 236–243. The article reviews the literature on the use of ECT in mental retardation, mostly with those diagnosed with 'psychotic depression'. Relapse occurred in half the recipients. See also Thuppal, M. & Fink, M. (1999). Electroconvulsive therapy and mental retardation. *Journal of Electroconvulsive Therapy, 15,* 140–149.
43. Wachtel, L. E., Dhossche, D. M. & Kellner, C. H. (2011). When is electroconvulsive therapy appropriate for children and adolescents? *Medical Hypotheses, 76* (3) 395–399; Wachtel, L., Griffin, M. & Reti, I. (2010). Electroconvulsive therapy in a man with autism experiencing severe depression, catatonia, and self-injury. *Journal of Electroconvulsive Therapy, 26* (1) 70–73.
44. Baeza, I., Flamarique, I., Garrido, J. M., Horga, G., Pons, A., Bernardo, M., Morer, A., Lázaro, M. L. & Castro-Fornieles, J. (2010). Clinical experience using electroconvulsive therapy in adolescents with schizophrenia spectrum disorders. *Journal of Child and Adolescent Psychopharmacology, 20* (3) 205–209.
45. Strober, M., Rao, U., DeAntonio, M., Liston, E., Amaya-Jackson, M., State, L. & Latz, S. (1998). Effects of electroconvulsive therapy in adolescents with severe endogenous depression resistant to pharmacotherapy. *Biological Psychiatry, 43,* 335–338.
46. Calev, A. (1994). Neuropsychology and ECT: Past and future research trends. *Psychopharmacological Bulletin, 30,* 461–469.
47. Parmar, R. (1993). Attitudes of child psychiatrists to electroconvulsive therapy. *Psychiatric Bulletin, 17,* 12–13.
48. Paillère-Martinot, M. L., Zivi, A. & Basquin, M. (1990). Utilisation de l'ECT chez l'adolescent. *Encéphale, 16* (5) 399–404.
49. Walter, G., Koster, K. & Rey, J. M. (1999). Electroconvulsive therapy in adolescents: Experience, knowledge, and attitude of recipients. *Journal of the American Academy of Child and Adolescent Psychiatry, 38,* 594–599.
50. Hale. E. (2009). Child shock therapy. Available at http://intcamp.wordpress.com/ect-kids/ (retrieved 8 September 2014).
51. Lima et al., 2013, p. 17. See note 35.
52. Jones, Y. & Baldwin, S. (1992). ECT: Shock, lies and psychiatry. *Changes: An International Journal of Psychology and Psychotherapy, 10* (2) 126–135, p. 134.
53. Collins, J., Halder, N. & Chaudhry, N. (2012). Use of ECT in patients with an intellectual disability: Review. *The Psychiatrist 36,* 55–60.
54. *Ibid.*
55. Aziz, M., Maixner, D. F., DeQuardo, J., Aldridge, A. & Tandon, R. (2001). ECT and mental retardation: A review and case reports. *Journal of Electroconvulsive Therapy, 17,* 149–152.
56. van Waarde, J. A., Stolker, J. J. & van der Mast, R. C. (2001). ECT in mental retardation: A review. *Journal of Electroconvulsive Therapy, 17,* 236–243.

57. ECT Statistics (2010). ECT use is not the same everywhere. Available at https://ectstatistics.wordpress.com/2010/08/19/ect-use-is-not-the-same-everywhere/ (retrieved 18 March 2015).
58. Mental Disability Rights International (2005). *Behind Closed Doors: Human rights abuses in the psychiatric facilities, orphanages and rehabilitation centers of Turkey.* MDRI. Available at www.youtube.com/watch?v=Q9INUsLLC8c (retrieved June 2015).
59. Herman, R. C., Dorwart, R. A., Hoover, C. W. & Brody, J. (1995). Variation in ECT use in the United States. *American Journal of Psychiatry, 152*, 869–875; Winslade, W., Liston, E. & Ross, J. (1984). Medical, judicial, and statutory regulations of ECT. *American Journal of Psychiatry, 141*, 1349–1355. This study compared the standards for ECT recommended by an APA taskforce report and those embodied in federal court orders and state statutes and regulations. The authors conclude that in spite of 'safeguards' promulgated by the psychiatric community, overregulation by legislatures and courts is commonplace. Legal standards can result in 'denials of service' while failing to resolve legal issues involving competence and consent.
60. Shorter, E. (2013). Electroconvulsive therapy in children. *How Everyone Became Depressed.* Available at http://www.psychologytoday.com/blog/how-everyone-became-depressed/201312/electroconvulsive-therapy-in-children (retrieved 5 August 2014).
61. Cassels, C. (2013). ECT in kids: Safe, effective, robust and... underutilized. Available at http://www.medscape.com/viewarticle/806923#3 (retrieved 5 August 2014).
62. APA (2013). The American Psychiatric Association's 2013 Annual Meeting. Abstract NR7-34. Presented 20 May 2013. Available at http://www.medscape.com/viewarticle/806923#3 (retrieved 5 August 2014).
63. Ibid.
64. Ibid.
65. Mangold, J. (Director) (2010). *Knight and Day* [film]. New York: 20th Century Fox.
66. Ghaziuddin, N., Kaza, M., Ghazi, N., King, C., Walter, G. & Rey, J. M. (2001). Electroconvulsive therapy for minors: Experiences and attitudes of child psychiatrists and psychologists. *Journal of Electroconvulsive therapy, 17*, 109–117.
67. Ross, C. A. (2006) The sham ECT literature: Implications for consent to ECT. *Ethical Human Psychology and Psychiatry, 8* (1) 17–28, p. 26.
68. Enns, M. W. & Reiss, J. P. (2015). Electroconvulsive therapy (Canadian Psychiatric Association Position Paper, published 16 March 2015). Available at https://ww1.cpa-apc.org/Publications/Position_Papers/Therapy.asp (retrieved 18 March 2015).
69. Ibid.
70. Ghaziuddin, N. & Walter, G. (Eds) (2013). *Electroconvulsive Therapy in Children and Adolescents.* Oxford: Oxford University Press.
71. Coffey, E. C. (1994). The role of structural brain imaging in ECT. *Psychopharmacology Bulletin, 3*, 477–483.
72. Ghaziuddin, N., King, C. A., Naylor, M. W., et al. (1996). Electroconvulsive treatment in adolescents with pharmacotherapy-refractory depression. *Journal of Child and Adolescent Psychopharmacology, 6* (4) 259–271.
73. Duckworth, K. (2009). National Alliance on Mental Illness: American Indian and Alaska Native women and depression FACT SHEET: What are the risk factors for American Indian and Alaskan Native women? Available at http://www2.nami.org/Template.cfm?Section=Women_and_Depression&Template=/ContentManagement/ContentDisplay.cfm&ContentID=88885 (retrieved 16 March 2015).
74. See, for example, Dillard, D. A., Smith, J. J., Ferucci, E. D. & Lanier, A. P. (2012). Depression prevalence and associated factors among Alaska native people: The Alaska Education and Research Towards Health (Earth) study. *Journal of Affective Disorders, 136* (3) 1088–1097.

75. Burstow, B. (2006). Electroshock as a form of violence against women. *Violence Against Women, 12* (4) 372–392.
76. Newnes, C. (2014). *Clinical Psychology: A critical examination.* Ross-on-Wye: PCCS Books, p. 146.
77. Editorial (1997). What is psychiatry? *American Journal of Psychiatry, 154* (5) 591–593, p. 593.
78. Lehmann, P. (2015). Securing human rights in the psychiatric field by utilizing advance directives. *Journal of Critical Psychology, Counselling and Psychotherapy, 15* (1) 1–10.
79. ABC News (2014). Electroshock therapy on under-14s banned in WA after law passes Parliament. Available at http://www.abc.net.au/news/2014-10-17/mental-health-bill-passes-wa-parliament/5822874 (retrieved 14 March 2015).
80. Aziz et al., 2001. See note 55.
81. Newnes, C. (2015). *Inscription, Diagnosis and Deception in the Mental Health Industry: How Psy governs us all.* Basingstoke: Palgrave Macmillan.

Chapter 10
Looking after children: Love, meaning and connection

Carolyn McQueen

The last two decades have seen a burgeoning interest in the problems faced by looked-after children. Whilst there are numerous positives associated with this there is the potential for children's sense of themselves to become obscured or lost in the maze of systems that are there to support them. In this chapter I reflect on some of the ideas that underpin the services and systems provided for looked-after children in the UK, and the impact of these on the identity and lives of children and young people who live away from their family of origin.

Context of current services

When a child is removed from their family of origin they enter a system of multiple agencies that seeks to protect and understand them. Within this system each agency has its own drivers and ideas which, whilst offering a diversity of perspectives around the child, also has the potential to create competing tensions as some narratives and ideas are introduced and taken up whilst others are discarded. These tensions play out throughout the child's time in care and can be pivotal in forming the young person's view of who they are.

The current wider sociopolitical context of the UK has shaped the strain between concern for this group of children and ideas about how best to meet their needs. Scandals such as Baby P and the sexual exploitation of young girls in Rotherham and Oxford caused outrage and disquiet in the UK. This public concern, particularly over Baby P, is believed to have been a major contributory factor that has fuelled the increase of children taken into care. The number of looked-after children in the UK at 31 March 2014 (31 July 2014 in Scotland) was 93,034, a rise from 88,083 in March 2010.[1,2,3,4] The main reason children were taken into care was abuse and neglect.

One effect of these rising numbers is to increase care costs at a time when local authority budgets are being cut and austerity is being promoted by the UK government as the way out of the recent economic crisis. In England in 2013/14 gross expenditure on looked-after children was estimated to be £2.5 billion. The majority of expenditure was on foster care services (55% of expenditure, around £1.4 billion, caring for 51,340 children and young people), and children's homes (36% of expenditure, around £0.9 billion, caring for 6,360 children and young people).[5] Estimates of the average social care cost per looked-after child range from £33,634 a year for children with no additional support needs to £109,178 for those with complex emotional or behavioural needs.[6]

Service guidelines advocate seamless interagency and partnership working to promote the emotional wellbeing of these children; yet NHS budgets are also being cut.[7] The House of Commons Health Committee Report on Child and Adolescent Mental Health Services (CAMHS) in England identified 'serious and deeply ingrained problems with the commissioning and provision of children's and adolescents' mental health services'.[8] The medical model continues to dominate children's mental health services and a holistic framework of children's emotional wellbeing is all too often subsumed as over-stretched and under-funded services focus their resources on children who meet the criteria for major psychiatric diagnoses such as depression, psychosis or eating disorders. Poor early care and nurture means that looked-after children often have attachment difficulties. For some, the levels of attachment problems are significant enough to meet the *DSM-5* criteria for reactive attachment disorder or disinhibited social engagement disorder. The association of attachment difficulties with mental health problems is complex; however, there is evidence that children with insecure attachment patterns are at greater risk of developing any mental health problem, though children with disorganised attachment patterns have the highest risk, particularly for externalising problems such as oppositional defiant disorder and conduct disorder.[9] Although more vulnerable to mental health problems, and often showing distinct clusters of problematic behaviours, looked-after children often fail to meet eligibility criteria for CAMHS.

Within this environment clinicians have looked to develop more innovative ways of providing services for looked-after children and young people. Ideas from neuroscience have been particularly influential in informing professionals' understanding of attachment theory and overall child development. Understanding the human brain and its development has come to be seen as the foundation to understanding human behaviour.[10] Advances in neuro-imaging have enabled the mapping of parts of the brain's development. The differences seen in children who have experienced early neglect and trauma, when compared with children who have not, have been used to formulate models of how the brain works and the impact on such children.[11,12,13] Practitioners have taken these findings and developed new interventions with looked-after children and their families.

This new wave of interventions has seen the focus move away from individual therapy with children towards the priority of providing a stable and secure home environment in which they can begin to feel safe.[14] Foster-carers are supported through consultations and training.[15] Sometimes there is work with the foster-carer and child together with the aim of promoting a more secure internal model of attachment in the child and helping them process trauma.[16,17]

My NHS post in Powys is funded by the local authority to work directly with carers and other professionals in the system. Similar service structures exist throughout the UK. The primary focus is on supporting carers to 'hold' the placement. This might involve offering strategies to manage a child's behaviour or help them process their feelings. Education about attachment and child development is offered, with the hope that carers will see the rationale for the strategies suggested and use them in their day-to-day parenting. Alongside this there is the more nebulous intervention: emotional support for the foster-carer. Difficult to define precisely or quantify, it is an important part of the process.

Keeping the family stable:
placement breakdown, meaning and connection

As a clinical psychologist who has worked with foster families for nearly 10 years I am interested in the meanings that carers and children make of their day-to-day lives together. Providing strategies is not necessarily the solution. Carers often feel they have 'done that' (and there was no change), or 'It won't work; he will just erupt.' Often they are at the end of their tether, faced with a child who expresses anger, sadness, fear in a multitude of ways, many of which challenge the family they find themselves living in. Over time this takes its toll on carers, and the initial enthusiasm and desire to nurture and 'make a difference' may fade. Caring and wanting to care become a burden. Professional explanations about brain function, arousal levels, or 'fight and flight' response become meaningless as the child's behaviour becomes perceived as personal – a rejection of the care that is offered. This often challenges the carers' sense of who they are. This is the point when placements are at high risk of breaking down.

Placement stability is associated with better social, emotional and educational outcomes for children.[18] Although services aim to create stable, long-term placements this doesn't always happen. Unplanned placement endings occur in approximately 19 to 40 per cent of foster-care placements.[19]

Placements break down for a host of reasons, only some of which relate to the child's immediate presentation: for example, the personal circumstances of the foster-carer, such as bereavement, chronic illness, ageing, divorce, etc. Factors correlated with placement breakdown include the child's age at placement, the number of previous placements, cognitive ability and educational achievement, level of mental health disturbance and a history of delinquency. Whereas most of us living in our own birth or chosen families would simply 'get on with it' (though not always easily), hopefully with a supportive community around us, all too often the looked-after child is unable to stay in placement and is moved. This may well be with little warning or choice. There still appears a reluctance to be open with children about moves and they may find themselves being picked up from school and driven to a new home, with little explanation or chance to say goodbye. What sense does the child make of the move and the aftermath? Or of the events that led up to it? How do they understand the wider system of 'care' around them? And how do these ideas influence their sense of who they are as children?

Foucault's ideas about knowledge and power provide a framework for understanding this.[20] Children in the looked-after system are subject to powerful narratives about who they are and who they should be. The nature of looked-after children means they are scrutinised and regulated by professionals in a way most children are not. When unchallenged this serves to define and shape their sense of self.

In modern Britain the whole discourse around care has come to imply a commodity that can be bought and provided in a mechanistic but exact way. For example, some of the recent revelations about carers for the elderly show that 15-minute slots are allocated in which to provide care.[21] That is not to say that the individual healthcare assistants do not care about the individuals they provide a service for; however, there is an objectified approach to care in a consumerist society, especially when cutbacks mean there is less money to provide services. Caring for others becomes a business where time and tasks are sold. Compassion and commitment are in danger of being secondary to the money that can be made. Although the term 'looked after' implies an emotional connection, that is, something beyond merely meeting the day-to-day physical needs of the child, for many of the children I meet it is alienating, a label that marks them as 'different' and visible to others.

For the child or young person, it may not feel as though 'caring' is involved in their experience of being 'looked after'. This is especially so when placements are beginning to break down. When foster-carers find they cannot care for a child, their sense of themselves as a 'carer' is often challenged and disrupted on a daily basis. It can become hard to hide feelings such as disappointment, failure and resentment from the child. For the child, there is confusion about their relationships with adults who are meant to 'care'. A placement that began with a mixture of hope and uncertainty becomes one where they experience themselves as unacceptable in some way and ultimately rejected. The interplay between a carer's sense of themselves and what they can offer and the child's sense of themselves creates powerful meanings for the child about who they are in relationship to others, both in the present and in the future.

Although the childhoods of many looked-after children have been marked by early trauma, separation and loss, they are far more complex. There are many constructions of childhood, each dependent on time, societal context, the child and the individuals involved in their life. For children who live away from their family of origin, loss, separation and trauma are a reality and provide dominant stories which are told and retold, and from which the children (and professionals around them) build meaning about their lives. Yet there are other realities which may be less attended to: moments when a child feels connected, understood or loved. What determines how much a child attends to these experiences? And is there a way the foster-carers, parents and professionals around the child can bring these to the fore?

Crafting new meanings

Individuals construct meaning from physical and emotional experiences and the ways that we relate to them. We interact with the world around us through our physical bodies, and our minds 'make sense' through language and ideas that are available to us at any given time. Neuroscience has provided knowledge on the complexities and two-way interactions between a child's environment and the developing brain. It gives explanations for why a child (or a parent) might have specific difficulties and provides a rationale to use specific strategies to help parent a child.[22] In my experience this way of understanding a child's behaviour helps foster-carers. It can release them from 'blaming' the child and allow them to adapt their care and use different approaches that focus more on providing stability and emotional nurturing. Yet what (if anything) does a focus on these ideas obscure?

A brain-based understanding of looked-after children focuses on the physical: that is, how our brains drive our caregiving impulses and how children's development is fundamentally affected by parent–child/carer–child interactions and leads to challenges and problems. It tells us very little about the meaning that foster-carers and children make of their situation. It is unsurprising that a science narrative dominates this area, given the predominance of the positivistic science model in our society. Yet clinicians do not just work with scientific reasoning; they are also faced with the broader and more complex meanings conferred by carers and young people. For example, a carer may understand that a child may become 'emotionally dys-regulated' because of a lack of soothing in early months, or that because of high anxiety and fear they find it hard to concentrate and learn in school. They may even, for a time, be able to use different ways to help the child calm down, or work with the school to make the environment feel safer; yet what enables them to continue to care and persist in providing a home for children over time? This is a core aspect of caring that clinicians and social workers have to work with as they support foster-carers. A carer may understand the scientific rationale of a behaviour whilst still deciding that they can no longer care for a child.

The research literature on looked-after children has centred mainly on the stresses and challenges faced by carers. This has been because of the correlation between carer stress and placement breakdown. Research findings have been used to develop interventions that support the foster-carer, particularly in understanding child development and attachment and providing practical strategies for parenting.

Recent studies have looked at positive outcomes in foster-care, and how particular qualities and characteristics of foster-carers are crucial to helping children and young people have a family life that is supportive and affirmative of them. These research studies draw on ideas from positive psychology, where the emphasis is on positive experiences, enduring psychological traits, positive relationships and positive institutions.[23]

These studies identified central themes that the foster-carers spoke of in their accounts of looking after the children. These included love and integration into the family.[24] The children were seen as part of the family and perceived as contributing positively to family dynamics. The carers described feelings of love and unconditional empathy for the child.

Other studies have identified the foster-carer commitment as a central component to successful placements.[25] When this construct was explored further with foster-carers who had had 'successful' placements (where successful was defined as having been in placement for at least two years, and in care for four years or more), individual carers spoke of being able to see a future relationship with the child; they had a sense of the child belonging in their family, whilst at the same time being able to both allow and promote the child's relationship with their family of origin.[26] As they constructed meaning about their ability to create and sustain a successful placement the carers spoke of tenacity and persistence in their care for the children, of being able to tolerate the ambiguous role as both a 'carer' and 'parent' to the child although the child has no commitment to them. They spoke of unconditional love for the child.

Carers who took part in these studies see themselves in a relationship with the children that is not merely 'professional' or a 'job'. There are narratives of commitment, love and attempts to understand the child. They provide rich descriptions of their roles, ones that include the child's birth family and how as carers they might navigate their way through the various tensions that emerge because of the unique position they hold in the child's life. Having these broader and complex meanings appears to have helped them persist in caring for and nurturing children in their care, despite any problems they encountered. Their feelings and accompanying actions create an experience for the child, where they are accepted and seen as something other than a challenge. In turn, these experiences form a space in which children can begin to feel cared for, a space in which they can belong. The dance between the foster-carers and the child becomes one of hope and enjoyment rather than endurance and challenge. The child's sense of who they are in relationship to others moves towards acceptance and love.

These qualitative research studies lend support to Hughes' PACE approach.[27] This advocates an attitude to parenting that incorporates **p**layfulness, **a**cceptance, **c**uriosity and **e**mpathy. There is an emphasis on a 'heart to heart' connection between the carer (parent) and the child. His model is strongly based on ideas of brain development and how care might become 'blocked' by neurobiology. From a social constructionist position, helping carers hold a position of playfulness, acceptance, curiosity and empathy towards a child frees them up to relate differently to the child. In so doing, there are new experiences of self and the potential for new meanings for both the carer and child – ones that are more affirmative, supportive and accepting.

Conclusion

Professionals working with looked-after children have greater knowledge than ever about children's development, neuroscience and child psychology. How do these ideas translate and transform the lives of looked-after children?

Historically, the concept of love has not been promoted in foster-care. Concerns about allegations against foster-carers or carers becoming 'too attached' have meant that qualities such as love and commitment have been separated from the role of the professional 'carer'. Yet these are the qualities that enable millions of families to survive and thrive day to day. By acknowledging these aspects of caring for children who do not live with their families of origin, professionals allow and support the potential for a deeper sense of connection between children and carers. This, in turn, creates space for the children to develop identities and relationships that are more affirming of their experience.

Endnotes

1. Department for Education (2014). Table A1. In *Children Looked After in England, Including Adoption: National tables* (XLSX). London: Department for Education.
2. Waugh, I. (2014). Section three: Looked-after children. In *Children's Social Care Statistics Northern Ireland 2013/14*. Belfast: Department of Health Social Services and Public Safety.
3. Scottish Government (2015). *Children's Social Work Statistics Scotland, 2013–2014*. Edinburgh: Scottish Government.
4. Stats Wales (2015). Children in need at 31 March by looked-after status, category of need and disability, including unborn children. Available at https://statswales.wales.gov.uk/Catalogue/Health-and-Social-Care/Social-Services/Childrens-Services/Children-in-Need/childrenneed-by-localauthority-categoryofneed (retrieved June 2015).
5. Harker, R. & Heath, S. (2014). *Children in Care in England: Statistics*. Standard Note SN/SG/4470. London: House of Commons Library.
6. Curtis, L. (2014). *Unit Costs of Health and Social Care 2014*. Canterbury: PSSRU.
7. Department for Education & Department of Health (2014). *Promoting the Health and Welfare of Looked-after Children: Statutory guidance for local authorities, clinical commissioning groups and NHS England*. London: DfE & DoH.
8. House of Commons Health Committee. (2014). *Children's and Adolescents' Mental Health and CAMHS: Third report of session 2014–15*. London: TSO, p. 3.
9. Solomon, J. & George, C. (2011). *Disorganized Attachment and Caregiving*. New York: Guilford Press.

10. Nelson, C. A., Fox, N. A. & Zeanah, C. H. (2014). *Romania's Abandoned Children: Deprivation, brain development, and the struggle for recovery.* Cambridge, MA: Harvard University Press.
11. Gerhardt, S. (2004). *Why Love Matters: How affection shapes a baby's brain.* Hove and New York: Brunner-Routledge.
12. Glaser, D. (2000). Child abuse and neglect and the brain: A review. *Journal of Child Psychology and Psychiatry, 41* (1) 97–116.
13. Schore, A. (2003). *Affect Dysregulation and Disorders of the Self.* New York: Norton.
14. Golding, K. S., Dent, H. R., Nissim, R. & Stott, L. (2006). *Thinking Psychologically About Children who are Looked After and Adopted: Space for reflection.* Chichester: Wiley.
15. Golding, K. (2003). Helping foster carers, helping children: Using attachment theory to guide practice. *Adoption and Fostering, 27* (2) 64–73.
16. Hughes, D. (2011). *Attachment-focused Family Therapy Workbook.* New York: Norton.
17. Booth, P. & Jernberg, A. M. (2010). *Theraplay: Helping parents and children build better relationships through attachment-based play* (3rd edition). London: John Wiley & Sons.
18. Kelly, G. & Gilligan, R. (2000). *Issues in Foster Care.* London: Jessica Kingsley.
19. Rushton, A. & Dance, C. (2004). The outcomes of late permanent placements: The adolescent years. *Adoption and Fostering, 28,* 49–58.
20. Foucault, M. (1977). *Discipline and Punish: The birth of the prison.* London: Penguin.
21. Leonard Cheshire Disability (2013). *Ending 15-minute Care.* Available at https://www.leonardcheshire.org/who-we-are/publications/latest-publications-download/ending-15-minute-care#.VYFWEsx8xaM (retrieved June 2015).
22. Hughes, D. A. & Baylin, J. (2012). *Brain-based Parenting: The neuroscience of caregiving for healthy attachment.* New York, NY: Norton.
23. Snyder, C. & Lopez, S. (2007). *Positive Psychology: The scientific and practical exploration of human strengths.* London: Sage Publications.
24. Taylor, S. (n.d.). *A Qualitative Exploration of Foster Carers' Positive Experiences.* Unpublished research thesis for the Doctorate in Clinical Psychology, Staffordshire and Keele Universities.
25. Dozier, M. (2005). *Attachment and Biobehavioral Catch-up: Infant Caregiver Project* [Unpublished manuscript]. Newark, DE: University of Delaware.
26. Oke, N., Rostill-Brookes, H. & Larkin, M. (2013, online 2011). Against the odds: Foster-carers' perceptions of family, commitment and belonging in successful placements. *Journal of Clinical Psychology and Psychiatry, 18,* 7–24.
27. Hughes, D. A. (2009). *Attachment-focused Parenting: Effective strategies to care for children.* New York: Norton.

Chapter 11

Don't blame the parents:
Is it possible to develop non-blaming models of parental causation of distress?

Rudi Dallos

Philip Larkin tells us, 'They fuck you up, your mum and dad.'[1] Referring to the quote, Alan Bennett remarked that, as a writer, if your parents in fact did not 'fuck you up' and were nice and stable, they left you with very little to write about so then they 'really fucked you up good and proper'. We have all been children and many of us have also become parents and so have seen the two sides of the coin: how exasperated, upset, angry, mad, crazy we can become about our parents; but also, as parents ourselves, how unfair it can seem that our children do not seem to appreciate what we have tried so hard to do for them, the sacrifices we have made, the money we have spent, the things we have given them that we never had … and so on.

Blame, guilt and forgiveness are arguably some of the most important concerns in family life. In my experience of working with families over 35 years, perhaps the most frequent and central issue in their lives together is that of blame and guilt. In a piece of 2006 research with families containing a young person with a diagnosis of anorexia we started by asking families to advise us:

RD: We are going to interview other families; what things do you think we should ask them? What would you be interested in us asking them?

Albert: ... we felt as though we were guilty. You, know, we didn't know what we'd done wrong if we were guilty and I wonder whether other people felt the same way ...

Guilt and blame appear to have been central to many of the families I have worked with clinically and in research. Where did we go wrong? It cannot be our fault – we tried so hard. Other parents have not been as good as us and yet their children are OK. It must be that she has an illness, anorexia, autism, ADHD, personality disorder, psychosis ... the labelling list goes on, and with each revision of the diagnostic manuals (*DSM-5*, *ICD-11*) seems to get longer. Like new stars, we keep discovering exotic new disorders. For example, *social anxiety disorder*, 'also known as social phobia, is an anxiety disorder involving discomfort around social interaction, and concern about being embarrassed and judged by others'.[2] This is in contrast to *disinhibited social engagement disorder*: 'a pattern of behavior in which a child actively approaches and interacts with unfamiliar adults.'[3] The first used to be called being a bit shy, and the second being very sociable. Of course extremes of such behaviours can be distressing and problematic for a child and their parents, but a central aim of this chapter is to illustrate how the sense of blame and failure drives many parents to embrace diagnostic labels which in the long term may be counterproductive and damaging to the family.

Core to such explanations are questions of causation, especially questions about why people act as they do – the issue of intention. How the question of intention is answered relates centrally to considerations of responsibility, approval and blame. It is important to distinguish the terms 'responsibility' and 'blame'. The former is invoked when we appear to have done something good, as well as bad: for example, developing a valued project or taking care of someone we recognise as being in need. Attribution theory suggests that people are more likely to claim responsibility (internal agency and causation) for successes and good actions but attribute failure to external causes.[4] Things are never quite so simple; people diagnosed as suffering with depression appear to find it harder to consider that they have achieved any success and instead may blame themselves for things they cannot possibly have caused, such as being abused as a young child by their parents.[5]

Michel Foucault argues that the explanations we employ in ascribing responsibility are embedded in a language located in our cultural histories of religious, scientific, artistic and legal discourses.[6] These discourses operate most powerfully when they are tacit, implicit and have the status of being taken for granted or 'common sense'. People have always been required to account for their actions. That which has been invoked as 'causal' varies. Religion has played a significant role by designating sinful or illegitimate action and thought that need to be accounted for, and which should rightfully lead to feelings of guilt and a search for forgiveness. Judeo-Christian ethics espouse the doctrine of original sin; for Roman Catholics a child is born flawed as a result of Adam and Eve's transgression in the Garden of Eden. Religious practice is required to cleanse this sin and to 'remove us from temptation'. In effect, bad behaviour is expected rather than requiring explanation. Instead 'goodness' has to be striven for by continual effort to resist Satan's temptations. Religious doctrine also posits that we could all fundamentally recognise good from evil, especially given appropriate guidance or religious schooling. The exceptions are some individuals seen as having been born evil who needed to be removed from society. In Roman Catholicism responsibility, guilt and seeking of forgiveness came to be embedded in the practice of the confessional. Importantly, confession consists in revealing actions, sinful thought *and* intentions. The confessional can also be seen as the prototype for psychotherapy, though psychotherapy obscures and disguises its moral premises. Psychotherapeutic concepts, such as neutrality, validation and an accepting stance, can be seen to reflect a New Testament ethic of forgiveness but with less clarity about *what* is to be forgiven.

Religious doctrine came to be embedded in canon law in which the Pope is the ultimate arbiter for morality and the content and framework of religious laws. This was developed into criminal law, eventually encapsulating the concept of responsibility as a central feature in judging culpability and due punishment. The question of intention behind actions was first addressed by the concept of *mens rea* (guilty mind). Influenced by canon law, *mens rea* entered into common law at the end of the twelfth century. This included more subtle considerations of whether an action was fully intended (for example, to deliberately harm or murder someone) or arose out of recklessness or lack of forethought (to be considered manslaughter in the case of causing death). Important considerations regarding the ability to understand or have a clear intention to act led to insanity or diminished responsibility as a mitigating plea for serious crime appearing in the late thirteenth century in English law.

Hippocrates (370 BCE) proposed that people varied in terms of their constitutions, being classifiable as melancholic, phlegmatic, sanguine or choleric, and that people's actions were shaped by their basic physiological dispositions. Responsibility for action is here not just located in our voluntary choices but also shaped by forces beyond our control – our natural temperaments. Attributions of responsibility are tempered with a consideration of the 'slings and arrows of outrageous fortune'. More subtly, this raises the idea that our choices of action are not simply or fundamentally personal, but contingent. As Marx said, 'We make choices but not in the circumstances of our own choosing.'[7]

This is a brief and cursory glance at some facets of responsibility.[8] In our research with families we find these themes repeatedly surfacing. Typical statements might include: 'He is doing it to wind us up' (voluntary choice), 'He was a "screamer" from the day he was born' (trait theory), 'I think he just fell in with the wrong crowd' (learning and social influence), and finally 'We think it is the attention deficit disorder.' The least overtly stated themes are explanations of responsibility as part of a mutual process, of the type 'We seem to be making things worse', or 'We're going round in circles.' Arguably such systemic conceptualisations are relatively recent to traditions of Western thought, in contrast to Eastern cultures and Buddhism. Systemic thinking and 'circular causality' – the view that we mutually influence each other and that unilateral influence, except in extreme cases, is a myth – have been a relatively new addition to Western thought and may still appear extraneous to 'common sense'.[9]

A family interaction: Carl had been adopted by Brenda and Mark when he was six years old, along with his younger brother Simon. His life in his family of origin had been very difficult and featured neglect, violence between his parents, alcoholism and violence towards him. The following dialogue took place during my personal research and clinical practice in 2014:

RD (to Mark –): Do you feel that sometimes he [Carl] thinks you don't care or don't love him?

Mark: I don't know ... I know that I am extremely p***ed off with him. Because it's eight years we have had him, seven years of absolute crap. [There are tears in his voice. Brenda touches his knee for comfort.] Police, police, running away, phoning social services, stealing, smoking, drinking, drugs dealing ... I've tried to talk to you. I'm peed off, unhappy. I love you. I don't think you want to be part of the family [tears in his voice] ... Take charge of yourself; otherwise you're gonna be on drugs, in jail and probably dead. And it ain't anything I can do. I'm angry [nodding head] ...

RD: Thanks for being honest.

Mark: I am honest. [Tearful] I just don't know what to do.

RD: Is it like this at home, that you have this conversation?

Mark: Yes, I am angry with him.

Carl: We don't really talk.

Mark: We don't talk, we don't do nothing.

Carl: I push people away …

Brenda: I don't know how much goes back to the early years … I was told he needs a strong male model. Wish I could get into his head … He needs me most when I'm angry with him [tears], when I'm angry with him, when he's done something wrong and I'm shouting; that's when I should be able to go to him … tell him he's wanted, but I can't do it, and I don't know how to do it, and I know I should.

This next passage illustrates how his adoptive parents now saw him as going off the tracks and that they also had a sense that he was rejecting them. They expressed that they were at their wits' end about what to do to help Carl, and that in fact wanting to help him was also tinged with anger at what they felt he was putting them through. Perhaps for adoptive parents some of the dilemmas are even sharper than they are for parents whose children are biologically theirs. Brenda and Mark appeared to feel that they had done it wrong and that they were to blame. For example, Brenda remarked that she did just the opposite of what she felt she *should* do, which was to show Carl love when he had done something wrong; instead she found herself angrily shouting at him. This was all very hard for Brenda and Mark to bear, given that they wanted to be kind in helping these disadvantaged young people. They had shown them more care and affection than their natural parents had; they had been thoughtful about the best ways to act, and had read psychological texts on parenting and taken advice from professionals – not least myself.

The outcome of this boiling pot of emotions, pain, hurt and anger can be a tendency to search for narratives which do not blame them so much: 'Maybe it all goes back to his early years,' 'Maybe it is his temperament' (bad blood), and, most compellingly for many families, 'Maybe he has a form of dysfunction or illness.' In Carl's case some candidates for labels might be personality disorder, sociopathic personality or ADHD. We should also note in the extract above that Carl himself starts to buy into diagnosis in his remark that 'I push people away,' implying perhaps that he thinks there is something wrong with him and there is little he can do to help this.

Models of parental responsibility

Why do parents typically feel blamed? There are a number of influential strands of research and explanations that now seem to be held in our collective consciousness as explicit forms of blaming of families for causing serious pathologies in their children. One is the model of anorexia proposed by Hilda Bruch, in which she described causal family environments characterised by overprotection, intrusiveness and control, with few opportunities for self-expression. She argued that these environments led to the development of a highly compliant 'false self' and self-starvation was a rebellion against such parental impingement. Anorexia was seen as a form of covert communication of protest and attempt for autonomy which typically emerged in adolescence.[10] Since the most central interaction was seen to be between the women in the family (90 per cent of those with anorexia are female), this model was experienced by many as gendered and as 'mother-blaming'. A similar model can be seen in Bateson's theory of schizophrenia. In this he argued that mothers engage in confusing and contradictory processes of communication with their children. At the verbal level a mother may say that she wants affection from her son but non-verbally expresses disgust. She also gives a message that this confusion must not be commented on since it might challenge the relationship and hurt her.[11] Bateson strongly implied that the ambivalent and contradictory communication arose out of a deep fear of potential rejection, and suggested in his description of 'double-bind' situations that these were driven by anxieties and insecurities:

> The *need of the mother to be wanted and loved* also prevents the child from gaining support from some other person in the environment, a teacher for example. A mother with these characteristics would feel threatened by any other attachment of the child and would sabotage any competing relationship in order to (break it up and) bring the child back closer to her with consequent *anxiety* when the child became *dependent* on her.[12] (Emphasis added)

As with Bruch's model, an unfortunate reaction to Bateson's theory was the impression that it was also mother-blaming. This view became so strongly established that it obscured later reformulations as a mutual and even a triadic process. It has been argued further that such patterns could be better seen as a triangular double-binding process, typically where the mother is or feels disempowered.[13] A third and perhaps even more powerful example comes from Kanner's theory of autism, which drew attention to what he saw as a lack of parental warmth and attachment to their autistic children. He attributed autism to a 'genuine lack of maternal warmth'. This led to the concept of the 'refrigerator mother'. (Kanner went on to describe the mothers of autistic children as 'just happening to defrost enough to produce a child'.[14]) His ideas have produced widespread criticism and now rejection by parents of children diagnosed with autism, people with the diagnosis and also professionals working with them. But it is very interesting to consider the arguments marshalled against his view, for example, that Kanner consistently ignored the fact that these children might have siblings who, despite living in the same family, do not have a diagnosis of autism. This would be a convincing argument were it not for the fact that it is also argued that autism is a genetically inherited condition, and that siblings, especially identical twins, are more likely to have the condition. The evidence seems to lie somewhere between these two positions – the evidence regarding identical twins is not convincing and does not support a genetic view, and there is evidence that other children in the family also show disturbances but not always enough to receive a diagnosis.

The purpose of paying attention to these models is not simply to attempt to justify them. Rather, I want to consider some broader implications for 'science' and clinical practice. What does all this feel like from 'inside' the family? I have worked clinically and conducted research interviews with families where a young person in the family was presenting with problems with eating – anorexia.[15] My experience of working with many of the families was of a very high level of anxiety in therapy and what felt like reluctance to talk about their relationships as in any way connected to the problem. I initially felt some irritation at what seemed like deliberate obstructiveness, but gradually developed a sense that the parents were doing their best but were struggling to draw on positive experience from their own childhoods. They also appeared to be terrified that they might have caused the problems. One 17-year-old, Cathy, perhaps captured (in what she says below) some of the parents' worst fears:

> The only thing I ever hear them talking about is me and if I didn't have this [anorexia] it's kind of like, would everything fall apart, at least it's keeping

> them talking. And they won't argue while I've got this because it might make me worse. So um ... that's kind of brought, sort of like, I'm not in control as such but I've got more control over the situation that way.

In this quote we hear the voice of a young woman who had been struggling with anorexia and whose family voluntarily agreed to engage in family therapy and research. What struck me in my work with them was that they were well-intentioned and wanted to understand what the problems were and how to resolve them. What was also impressive was that they knew about the dominant discourses of anorexia as a medical 'illness' but were not satisfied that there was not more to it than this, and that, as parents, they had got some things wrong. In an individual interview Cathy's father Albert said, 'We used to argue a lot [he and his wife] when Cathy was young and she used to hear it, and it upset her ... I think maybe we have come to pay a price for that?'

Family therapy has been around for over 50 years and during that time there have been some dramatic changes – not least that many therapists have become uncomfortable with the term 'family therapy'. One of the reasons for this is that the term appears to imply that parents are to blame for the problems and distress manifested in their children. This unease has also been fuelled by various parent groups who have reacted strongly to research and clinical practice which have appeared to suggest, as described earlier, that problems such as anorexia are 'caused' by problematic forms of family transactional processes.

Similar suggestions were being made about family life by John Bowlby, who described types of communicational and emotional processes in families that could lead to severe and complex attachment insecurity and problem development. He talked about the processes in families regarding children's experiences – 'On knowing what you are not supposed to know and feeling what you are not supposed to feel' – where children 'forget' significant distressing and painful events because their parents persuade or even coerce them into doing so.[16] Like R.D. Laing, Bowlby noted that in many cases parents encourage children to forget painful episodes in the genuine belief that this will somehow protect their child's sanity.[17] Despite their intentions being benign, such distortion could lead children to experience confusion, insecurity and a fragmented sense of self and reality. Bateson, Bowlby and Laing all shared a belief that families need to be able to engage in open and undistorted communicational transactions, and that significant problems arise when patterns of distortion, deception and denial become central to the family's functioning.

Dyads and families

A possible confusion that has arisen in considering family causation is that it has been seen as synonymous with a dyadic perspective and specifically as mother-blaming. In all of the above examples the central dynamics were regarded to be between the mother and a child. But a view of family systems as related to problems is broader than this. The fundamental unit of analysis is seen to be triadic: typically the parents and the child. The idea of children as becoming entangled in their parents' distress and conflicts has been central to family therapy. The research has lagged behind clinical intervention and a focus on 'triangulation': the process whereby a child can be destructively drawn into the parents' conflicts. Recent research does support the view that triadic conflicts can relate to the aetiology of problems in children.[18] A triadic formulation is not blaming any one person in a family, though it can still be experienced as blaming of the parents. Systemic perspectives strongly advocate a stance of neutrality, such that in triadic processes no one is to blame and all play a part in maintaining the processes. Despite this, it is of course tempting to think that there are fundamental inequalities in how much parents (as opposed to an infant) can construct the family relational system.

The dynamics of labelling: costs and benefits

Parents, as in the examples above, can be extremely distressed at the implication that they have caused serious problems to develop in their children. Albert indicated regret that marital conflicts may have negatively impacted on his daughter. Given the pervasiveness of medical models of problems such as anorexia it is then very compelling for parents to turn to illness labels to alleviate their sense of blame. This has been extensively discussed as one of the beneficial effects of an illness diagnosis.[19] Alongside the sense of relief for the parents can be a related 'closure' whereby alternative and family related explanations are eliminated.[20] But this process also involves the young person in the family:

Albert: You know, we didn't know what we'd done wrong, if we were guilty, and I wonder whether other people felt the same way …

Mary: … That's the way you do feel. You stop and think, is it what we did?

Cathy: They didn't make you feel guilty though, you felt guilty.

Albert: Well, some of the questions made you feel guilty …

Cathy: When I was in hospital one of the nurses was telling me that someone they had in there was diagnosed as anorexic and then when they did a brain scan she had a tumour on part of her brain and once they took it away she was eating normally. And the nurse who was talking to me reckons that proves it's just something in your brain.

This passage illustrates how the parents may feel a sense of preoccupying blame for having caused their daughter's 'anorexia' and that they also feel that professionals are implying this in their questions. Cathy, appearing to sense her parents' distress, steps into this process to tell the story of a tumour as appearing to have caused anorexia. In supporting this view she can be seen to be protecting her parents.

But the process also goes further than this. An illness diagnosis also protects Cathy from an implication that she is to blame:

RD: Looking back, what were your memories of mealtimes?

Cathy: Um, when I was very young I hated them, really. I was so fussy. I used to give most of it to the cat … very fussy … I can only remember one roast dinner which I was so annoyed to have to go to because I was playing outside and I would prefer to be playing than eating that and then I'd be left there with, 'You've gotta eat your meat.' And everyone would be on my back with, 'Oh you've gotta eat your greens' … I was so fussy wasn't I?

An alternative to an illness label may be the implication that a child is wilfully manipulative, destructive, difficult and causing problems in the family. This can be accompanied by a discourse that it is related to personality traits – as above, of being 'fussy'. Cathy in the extract checks for confirmation about this with her parents, that she really was 'fussy'. This position, through taking away some of the blame from the parents, also places it back on Cathy. Families can be seen to be caught in a Catch-22 dilemma: blaming themselves is painful, but an alternative, blaming their daughter, is also painful. One possible reaction of professionals – in wanting to absolve both parties from blame – is the notion that it is an illness. Now no one is blamed: it is an illness.

Coulter and Rapley add an important layer to these explorations of the role of families in the construction of distress and problems. They suggest that parents may also be caught in a trap whereby a significant body of government policy and legislation clearly implies that parents hold 'moral responsibility' for the behaviour of their children. Contemporary legislation, for example, assumes notions of some parents as feckless and irresponsible, and as the cause of a variety of deviant and dangerous behaviours in the children. This has included the use of parenting orders in cases where children act in unruly and antisocial ways. These political initiatives and policies clearly set a context whereby parents are made to feel responsible. Coulter and Rapley go on to argue that, 'Paradoxically, whereas the laity view the actions of parents as being instrumental in the emotional development of their children, some commentators suggest that it is, for the psy(chotherapy) professions, now a prohibited topic' (my italics).[21]

The identification of the apparent contrast between common, lay explanations of mental health problems and their causes, and the shyness of the psychotherapy professions to address the question of the role of families in the causation of problems, adds an important layer of analysis to family therapy. There arose a powerful backlash in the 1970s against research which, for example, indicated that family dynamics had an important role in the genesis of madness and distress.[22] Research psychologists and psychiatrists subsequently have had to tread a fine line to avoid lawsuits from family rights groups and the support that these movements received from the pharmaceutical industry and mainstream medically oriented psychiatry.

At the core of the discussion about the role of family dynamics run some very important dilemmas and complexities, easily obscured by emotions generated by the issues involved. One consequence Coulter and Rapley suggest is the move to a vulnerability–stress model, for example of psychosis, which emphasises causation in terms of an individual 'biogenetic vulnerability' triggered by stress and conflict.[23] As such, families are not implicated in causing the symptoms but as possibly aggravating the problems, in part because the 'illness' causes the family members so much tension and distress. Treatment consequently features sympathising with the parents, regarding the 'illness' as a lifelong disability that they are struggling to cope with, and supporting and 'educating' them to be able to act in less critical and emotionally aroused ways.[24]

Coulter and Rapley describe how families appear to position themselves within these competing accounts: the lay views stressing their responsibility and the psychotherapy professions emphasising individual vulnerability and exoneration of the family. They also remind us that where parents are clearly seen to be engaging in physically or sexually 'abusive' or irresponsible behaviours to produce antisocial children, the question of responsibility clearly falls to the parents as culpable:

> In instances of unequivocal and deliberate abuse, where their behaviour self-evidently contravenes common sense understanding of the 'moral duties' that parents have towards their children, professional blaming of the parents appears unproblematic. Yet in circumstances without apparent gross violation, where the moral status of the parents' actions is not obvious ... while Psy may be incoherent about parental responsibility, parents are not.[25]

Coulter and Rapley offer examples of conversations with families where they indicate that the parents are fully aware of the dominant lay views of parental responsibility but employ a variety of strategies to soften the sense of self-blame that common lay opinion appears to hold. For example, they describe a key strategy, directly connected to avoiding this contradiction between lay and Psy perspectives, of stating that since they are not experts they do not know what caused their child's problems. In this they avoid absorbing the lay moral positions of responsibility and potential blame for their child's psychosis, and bow to professional knowledge which is in fact more unsure of the parents' role in causation and more likely to hold individualistic, illness interpretations.

As always, there can be a danger in such discussions of appearing antagonistic to families. This is not intended in this chapter and, on the contrary, it needs to be noted and applauded (given these dilemmas for families) how remarkable it is that, not only do they agree to participate in family therapy when directed to do so, but also that many families voluntarily seek family therapy. This suggests that despite the dominant views of the Psy profession, which favour a medical diagnosis, many parents actively resist this process and the attendant labelling of their child. They show a courageous resistance to the dominant medical discourse and are willing to consider that they may have some responsibility. They are further willing to consider ways of changing their relationships with each other in the hope that it will help their child. I frequently feel humbled by the courage of parents and their commitment to assisting their children by engaging in an enterprise in which they may feel potentially blamed and criticised, despite the reassurance of therapists that family therapy does not involve blaming. Many parents still have an 'open mind' about causation and have turned towards possible medical explanations out of desperation as a last ditch resort because no one has been able to advise what else might be helpful.

McHoul and Rapley illustrate how parents, in conversations with a paediatrician about their child's possible ADHD, attempted at many points to introduce a consideration of non-medical explanations, such as social issues at school or family dynamics, but were subtly directed back to a medical framework and the potential benefits of medication. They describe, for example, how parents' descriptions of normal siblings' rivalries as potentially contributing to some aspects of difficult behaviours could be largely ignored, and eventually the conversation steered towards a discourse of trying medication as a sort of trial or experiment:

Fa: He idolises his brother and I think part of it, he may be trying to be like his brother.

Dr: Mm hm.

Fa: But he doesn't ha – hasn't got the guts to do a lotta the stuff his brother does.

Dr: Mm hm.

Fa: Chickens out …

Dr: Well I mean I'd certainly make the diagnosis 'v er, ADHD based on the questionnaires plus … um … you know observations in the class but – uhmn and give him a trial of medication and we'll see what happens if …[26]

We have to be careful not to slip too easily into 'blaming' medical practitioners, especially in that they too often have positive intentions to be helpful to distressed parents. In this light Coulter and Rapley remind us that there are more profound contradictions and dilemmas in play, and suggest that one of the central considerations here is the subtle difference between responsibility and blame.[27] Critical to drawing a difference here is the issue of intention – so that contemplating parental involvement in the genesis of conduct does not necessarily imply the intent to cause it. This can help to 'offer a way out of the current reliance on neither a simplistic illness-blaming model that says it's not at all their fault, or an equally simplistic family-blaming model that says it's all their fault'.[28]

Corrective and replicative scripts

In Coulter and Rapley's research on family conversations relating to psychosis they noted that parents typically attempted to frame their intentions as positive. This can helpfully connect with a more compassionate account of how families may try to do the best they can but also do things that can cause distress and problems. Similarly, Bowlby has suggested that many parents believe that it is better for the child in his or her best interest to ignore or even to pretend that some things have not happened.[29] The question of intention is perhaps paramount in this discussion. But as the wise if pessimistic proverb states: 'The road to hell is paved with good intentions.' John Byng-Hall has articulated the idea of corrective and replicative scripts as underpinning transgenerational processes in families.[30] A corrective script is defined as the parents' intention to do things differently to and better than their own parents. Importantly, this idea emphasises that parents generally have positive intentions. Parents may describe trying to be more emotionally available for their children than their parents had been, to enforce less strict rules and discipline, or to foster validation and encouragement of their children's abilities. Likewise, they may hold an intention to repeat what they see as having been positive aspects of their own experience of being parents. These scripts may not be conscious but generally parents are able, with some prompting, to articulate their ideas about what they want to do differently.

The idea of corrective scripts both allows us to recognise parents' positive intentions and also offers an important clue as to why it is so difficult to ask them to consider responsibility and why they are more likely to feel blame. Given that many parents have struggled hard in trying to overcome adversity that they may have experienced as children, it can be doubly disappointing and appear grossly 'unfair' that they should feel to blame for having caused problems for their own children. It is possible that the more severe the adversity the parents have suffered in their own childhoods the more proud they may be that they have been able to survive. To consider that despite their best efforts they have nevertheless contributed to their child's distress and problems may seem unbearable to contemplate. In fact this dilemma may be problematic not only for parents but also for therapists and others working with families. We want to hold an optimistic view of life, which is that people do have natural capacities for healing and growth. An example is the development of the post-traumatic growth movement which focuses on the potential not just to overcome but actually to grow from difficult, potentially traumatic experiences.[31]

We are not simply or predominantly rational. Many of our actions and decisions are shaped by unconscious forces outside of our awareness.

Arguably most models of therapy and aetiology at least partly include this view. Our experiences and decision-making can be seen to occur at interconnected layers of representations: procedural, sensory, semantic, episodic and integrative.[32] Our earliest experiences prior to language are held as embodied representation of experience. For example, in relation to procedural memory my body remembers (in a similar way that it remembers how to ride a bicycle) that when I was frightened as a child and sought comfort from my mother or father, they became tense and awkward about touching or soothing me. Now when I am with my own children I may have a conscious (semantic) corrective script that I want to be emotionally available to and give comfort to my children. These rational, semantic intentions are not always so easily translated into behaviour. We may find ourselves, despite our intentions, also withdrawing as our parents did. One suggested narrative (or reason) for this is that children who have experienced a 'secure' attachment relationship with their parent have experienced not just the parent being available but also how the parent has corrected or repaired times when unable to be caring or when they are busy, distracted and so on. These processes of sophisticated adjustments and repair give a broader and more stable sense that our parents will be available. But without this experience the parents attempting a corrective script may try to be constantly available for their child – a draining and virtually impossible option. They may then feel that they have failed when they cannot achieve their unrealistic expectations and may consequently try harder, possibly intruding into their child's actions and generating anxiety. Alternatively they may feel depressed and withdraw. Cathy described above how she wanted to play when her mother made Sunday meals. However, such mealtimes were important to her mother because she wanted to correct the depressing, sad time that she had experienced with her own mother, who had suffered in ways described as depressed through most of her childhood. Many young women struggling with anorexia have described similar experiences of trying to be grateful to a mother who was desperate to cook for them and who wanted to be valued as a good mother.

This is the downside to corrective scripts. They can, in effect, set parents up to fail by not being able to achieve the extremely high standards they are setting themselves. Further to this, parents who have experienced highly dangerous events which have led them to feeling traumatised may develop extremely rigid and inflexible corrective scripts. Their interactions with their own children may trigger powerful procedural and sensory memories, such that the drive to be different (corrective script) becomes compulsive. It is not uncommon to hear some parents say they do not want to do anything the same as their parents. This can become a drive serving to obscure their responses to feedback from their children about how they are experiencing their parenting; in effect it can short-circuit feedback in their interactions. My experience has been that helping parents to become aware of this can be helpful. It can take some considerable time before they are able to surface from the anxiety of feeling blamed and be able to consider such processes. An important ingredient is that they are able to feel safe in the therapeutic situation and trust that the therapist is not intending to blame them.

The processes 'inside' families are also influenced by wider cultural expectations, so that attempts to 'do things better' need to be seen in the context of what parents understand to be 'better' and also what constitutes a problem. Coulter and Rapley point out that parents may find themselves caught between lay views that they are responsible and can and should do something to assist their children's problems, in contrast to Psy professionals' views that they are not responsible. Perhaps nowhere is this a more marked contradiction than in the realm of family therapy. Family therapists try to find ways to resolve this dilemma: for example, by adopting a non-blaming stance whilst at the same time considering alternatives and how family conflicts may be related to the problems. But there can be a sort of cat and mouse game where the issue of responsibility is not explicitly identified and named, running the risk that as a consequence the relationship with the family becomes inauthentic. This is perhaps most apparent in that family therapy teams will sometimes speak in exasperation after a family has left about how they see parents acting in destructive and unhelpful ways, but without voicing this to the families themselves.

Responsibility versus blame

Writing this chapter it is also important to reflect on my own position. Why am I interested in this topic? Perhaps it is because I am still angry at my own parents? This is partly true and I think in part I still want to express my protest and hurt at what I perceive to be my own parents' unavailability, the demands they have made on me and the anxieties they have 'caused' me. I have likewise heard children in my clinical practice express that they want a simple apology or acknowledgement from their parents rather than excuses or avoidance. It would be a simple solution though if an apology from our parents was enough. Perhaps this can be helpful but it is more complex than this and frequently when parents do apologise this can also trigger mixed emotions in a child, leading them to feel responsible, guilty and to blame themselves. It is very tempting to attempt to resolve these contradictory feelings by turning to the simplicity of an illness discourse.

Bowlby has suggested that a therapist becomes a transitional attachment figure for family members, and an important aspect of becoming a potential source of security and trust for the family is that she or he will also be subject to their vulnerability and anger.[33] As we have seen, part of this vulnerability is a sense that they have failed. But in the examples that I have considered above, the parents have not failed. Even in cases of extreme problems there are often still many features of a child that can be seen as positive and 'normal' versus pathological. A useful exercise can be to map the territory and influence of the 'illness'. For example, in my recent work with a family with a seven-year-old girl with a diagnosis of autism, I asked her to draw two overlapping pictures of herself and colour in how much of her was autism and how much her normal self. She said, 'My hands, arms, legs and eyes are not autistic but my mouth and my brain is.' Then we drew how much of her brain was not autistic and she explained that dreaming and reading were not but sometimes speaking and interacting with others were. She also mentioned that the balance between her normal self and autistic self varied at different times and places, for example, that the autistic self was more at school and less at home.

Hopefully, this activity and others like it can help families to explore their understandings; nevertheless it is very likely that, as the mother listened to her daughter talking, feelings of anxiety may have arisen for her. Most likely such a questioning could imply that it was not really an illness and hence was her fault. It is then extremely compelling to offer reassurance that we believe it is an illness and not caused by parenting. Though it can be difficult it may be more helpful to explore these feelings of guilt and responsibility. In fact it is often the first thing that families want to talk about but it often ends up as the last or is completely avoided.

Endnotes

1. Larkin, P. (1971). This be the verse. In Farrar, Straus and Giroux (Eds) (2001). *Collected Poems*. London: Faber and Faber.

2. Grohol, J. (2013). Symptoms of disinhibited social engagement disorder. Psych Central. Available at http://psychcentral.com/disorders/symptoms-of-disinhibited-social-engagement-disorder/ (Retrieved 5 January 2015).
3. Ibid.
4. Kelley, H. H. (1967). Attribution theory in social psychology. *Nebraska Symposium on Motivation*, *15*, 192–238.
5. Bateson, G. (1972). *Steps to an Ecology of Mind.* New York: Ballantine.
6. Foucault, M. (1967). *Madness and Civilisation: A history of insanity in the age of reason.* London: Tavistock.
7. Marx, K. & Engels, F. (1846/1970). *The German Ideology* (Ed. C. J. Arthur). New York: International Publishers.
8. For a further analysis of 'responsibility' see Baker, E. & Newnes, C. (2005). The discourse of responsibility. In C. Newnes & N. Radcliffe (Eds). *Making and Breaking Children's Lives.* Ross-on-Wye: PCCS Books, pp. 30–40.
9. Ugazio, V., Fellin, L., Pennacchio, R., Negri, A. & Colciago, F. (2012). Is systemic thinking really extraneous to common sense? *Journal of Family Therapy*, *34* (1) 53–71.
10. Bruch, H. (1973). *Eating Disorders: Obesity and anorexia and the person within.* New York: Basic Books; Bruch, H. (1980). Preconditions for the development of anorexia nervosa. *American Journal of Psychoanalysis*, 40, 169–172.
11. Bateson, G., Jackson, D. D., Haley, J. & Weakland, J. H. (1956). Toward a theory of schizophrenia. *Behavioral Science*, *1* (4) 251–264.
12. Ibid. p. 251.
13. Weakland, J. (1976). Toward a theory of schizophrenia. In C. E. Sluzki & D. D. Ransom (Eds) (1976). *Double Bind: The foundation of the communicational approach to the family.* New York: Grune and Stratton.
14. Kanner, L. & Eisenberg, L. (1956). Early infantile autism 1943–1955. *American Journal of Orthopsychiatry*, *26* (3) 556–566.
15. Dallos, R. & Denford, S. (2008). A qualitative exploration of relationship and attachment themes in families with an eating disorder. *Clinical Child Psychology and Psychiatry*, *13* (2) 305–322.
16. Bowlby, J. (1988). *A Secure Base.* New York: Basic Books.
17. Laing, R. D. & Esterson, A. (1964). *Sanity, Madness and the Family.* London: Tavistock.
18. Dubois-Comtois, K. & Moss, E. (2008). Beyond the dyad: Do family interactions influence children's attachment representations in middle childhood? *Attachment & Human Development*, *10* (4) 415–431; Dallos, R., Lakus, K., Cahart, M. & McKenzie, R. (2015, in press). Becoming invisible: The effect of triangulation on children's well-being. *Clinical Child Psychology and Psychiatry.*
19. Grunebaum, H. & Chasin, R. (1978). Relabeling and reframing reconsidered: The beneficial effects of a pathological label. *Family Process*, *17* (4) 449–455.
20. Klainman, A. (1988). *The Illness Narratives: Suffering, healing, and the human condition.* New York: Basic Books; Crix, D., Stedmon, J., Smart, C. & Dallos, R. (2012). Knowing 'ME' knowing you: The discursive negotiation of contested illness within a family. *Journal of Depression and Anxiety*, *1*, 119, doi: 10.4172/2167-1044.1000119.
21. Coulter, C. & Rapley, M. (2011). 'I'm just, you know, Joe Bloggs.' In M. Rapley, J. Moncrieff & J. Dillon (Eds). *De-Medicalizing Misery.* London: Palgrave Macmillan, p. 160.
22. Weakland, 1976. See note 13.
23. Coulter & Rapley, 2011. See note 21.
24. Leff, J. & Vaughn, C. (1985). *Expressed Emotion in Families: Its significance for mental illness.* New York: Guilford Press.

25. Coulter & Rapley, 2011, p. 172. See note 21.
26. McHoul, A. & Rapley, M. (2005). A case of attention-deficit/hyperactivity disorder diagnosis: Sir Karl and Francis B. slug it out on the consulting room floor. *Discourse and Society, 16* (3) 419–449.
27. Coulter & Rapley, 2011. See note 21.
28. Read, J. & Gumley, A. (2008). Can attachment theory help explain the relationship between childhood adversity and psychosis? *Attachment: New directions in psychotherapy and relational psychoanalysis, 2* (1) 1–35; Read, J., van Os, J., Morrison, A. & Ross, C. (2005). Childhood trauma, psychosis and schizophrenia: A literature review with theoretical and clinical implications. *Acta Psychiatrica Scandinavica, 112,* 330–350.
29. Bowlby, 1988. See note 16.
30. Byng-Hall, J. (1995). *Rewriting Family Scripts: Improvisations and systems change.* New York: Guilford Press.
31. Seligman, M. E. P. & Csikszentmihalyi, M. (2000). Positive psychology: An introduction. *American Psychologist, 55* (1) 5–14.
32. Bowlby, 1988. See note 16; Crittenden, P. M. (2006). A dynamic-maturational model of attachment. *Australian and New Zealand Journal of Family Therapy, 27,* 105–115; Schacter, D. L. & Tulving, E. (Eds) (1994). *Memory Systems.* Cambridge, MA: MIT Press.
33. Bowlby, 1988. See note 16.

Chapter 12

The children's disability living allowance form: Policing dependency with a boundary object

Orly Klein and Carl Walker

Disability living allowance (DLA) is a non-means-tested, non-contributory UK benefit introduced in 1992. The children's DLA award is designated to help carers and parents to cope with the extra costs of looking after a child with complex needs, and it has both a care and a mobility component. Recent research has suggested that there is a lack of both official data and formal debate about the effectiveness of the UK system of deciding and monitoring claims for DLA in children. Banks and Lawrence have suggested that there is significant under-application for children's DLA and that children in disadvantaged families are less likely to apply for, and less likely to receive, a DLA award. Many who are eligible do not claim and it has been suggested that there are inconsistencies in award-making for those who do. Significantly, 97.3 per cent of their respondents reported finding the form difficult to complete.[1]

This is important since, on average, families with disabled children face three times the costs that other parents do, due to the likes of special diets, travel, clothing and heating. In addition to this, a chronic lack of affordable and suitable childcare means that many such parents are excluded from the labour market, mothers disproportionately so.[2,3,4,5] Steyn et al. note, therefore, that DLA offers a vital source of financial assistance for many.[6]

Drawing on the experiences of parents of children with additional needs in south-east England, this chapter draws upon Star's and Star and Griesemer's concept of the 'boundary object' to explore in detail the process of completing the children's DLA form.[7,8] In so doing we will unpack the key problems in children's DLA application and awards outlined above.

The DLA form as a boundary object

In exploring the general principles of welfare allocation, Langan suggests that an array of forms and questionnaires has been used to allocate individuals to a number of predetermined dependency categories in order to establish levels of priority.[9] However, all authorities have struggled both with the formulation and consistent application of eligibility criteria. Moreover, and crucially for this analysis, many people find it a particularly onerous challenge to identify, quantify, articulate and assert their needs. Furthermore, it is questionable whether the gap between the meaning that care regimes can have for the people who live them, and the semantic reduction that any form entails, allows for a sufficiently meaningful representation of such complex, varying and multifaceted regimes of care. Fassin and d'Halluin, speaking of the use of medical certificates to register the torture experiences of asylum seekers, noted how such forms, in reifying the asylum seekers' past experiences, are inevitably detached from the lived experiences of the victims of persecution, and the attempted objectification inevitably ends up de-subjectifying them.[10]

Valle and Aponte's study of parents' interactions with school professionals highlighted the routine disqualification of parents' voices in this arena, and went on to note that once children are captured in written documents, this becomes the truth by which all other interpretations are measured.[11] Moreover, this truth becomes completely dependent on the protocols through which the body and mind of the person are being read.[12]

Berg notes that technologies such as welfare application forms are inherently social in the sense that they play a core role in the lives of the people who use them.[13] Such forms provide an object through which assessors can chart, discuss and compare different social territories, and they exist to provide representations of lived experiences. In so doing, comparisons within and between people are facilitated through and reified by the structure of the form itself. But while such forms may be scrupulously deliberated in the design phase, they invariably manifest unforeseen impacts and consequences. Indeed, this chapter highlights some of these consequences for the parents of children with additional needs.

Star conceptualised 'boundary objects' as objects that people act toward or with. These are objects that reside between different social worlds and allow a degree of cooperative work on the absence of either consensus or indeed a forum for the development of consensus.[14] Boundary objects are objects that are used in different ways by different communities and act as a means of translation. As such, they facilitate a degree of translation across intersecting but largely separate social worlds. Typically they form the boundaries between groups.

For these reasons we argue there may be value in regarding the children's DLA form as a boundary object that exists between the parents who are making a claim for financial support and the government agencies tasked with measuring, standardising and rewarding various but specific regimes of parent-carer work: to collect, coordinate and distribute forms of knowledge about children and their families. Conceptualised as a boundary object, the children's DLA form is effectively an instrument of governance, a technology used to render caring regimes knowable and rewardable in specific ways. The form has the effect of shaping how the lives of families seeking financial support for their child with complex needs are rendered knowable, and quantifying the extent to which their suffering has value. Where the concept of boundary object brings purchase to the analytic framework in this chapter is that it allows the DLA form not only to be framed as a tool of translation between very different communities with very different needs, but it also provides a way to examine the impact of this translational bureaucracy on the lives of the parents who seek support.

A politics of expertise

It should be noted that a focus on the children's DLA form as a technical tool for translating experience requires consideration within a specific socioeconomic milieu. Claims on the state for financial support of any nature, and the bureaucracies mobilised to determine the validity of such claims, have for a number of years been subject to what Fassin and d'Halluin and Das call a 'Politics of Suspicion'.[15,16] Such claims run counter to neoliberal inclinations to construct modern subjects as self-regulators capable of managing and overcoming the vicissitudes of modern life.[17] These discourses have configured the neoliberal subject as an autonomous agent who should be both capable of and motivated to narrate their life stories. And, just as Fassin and d'Halluin note how the medical certificate that reifies previous experiences of torture enacted upon asylum seekers was particularly welcome in such a climate of suspicion, so DLA forms are similarly welcome. Although not completed by agents assumed to be neutral and authoritative, they are scrutinised by such agents and, as such, guard against anxieties of fraudulent dependency on the state. In so doing they provide a means through which to distinguish the more deserving from the less deserving and to further distinguish both of these from those who deserve no state support at all.

What is notable about the children's DLA form is that it appears to be the one form of contact with state apparatuses where parental judgement, expertise and knowledge are considered sufficiently substantial to use as the basis for potential government activity. Valle and Aponte have noted how the social relations between the parents of children with additional needs and professionals – usually medical professionals, teachers and SENCOs (special educational needs coordinators) – are often problematic.[18] Since parents are adjudged as being unable to bring the requisite objectivity necessary for the management of their children, and because they don't have access to privileged expert knowledge and professional discourses, they can experience a marginalisation and denigration of their knowledge. Parents find their knowledge subjugated and disqualified because they do not carry the authority of scientificity.[19] As such, parents are often assigned walk-on roles when they enter these specialised arenas, where they try to engage with the specialised languages of science, law, education and medicine, from which they are often deliberately excluded.[20] Here they come to learn that education and medical professionals have the authority to direct and terminate discourse; they come to hear their child described as an amalgamation of test scores, discrepancies, deficits and limitations, and feel patronised and/or at the mercy of professionals, who enact the conversations of deficit from which they are excluded.[21]

Many parents feel that they are expected to comply with professionals rather than engage in open discussion, and dosReis et al. noted that 21 per cent of healthcare professionals and school personnel were considered dismissive of parental concerns.[22,23] It has been suggested that the prevalent view of families of children with additional needs is that they are deficient and conflictual and evidence chronic sorrow, and that this persists among many healthcare professionals.[24] Indeed paediatricians frequently rate families as more distressed than parents do, with a focus on their supposed depression, poor parenting skills, family conflict and marital trouble. As a result of these widespread and erroneous beliefs regarding family conflict and parenting skills – of being seen as being handicapped by an incapacity to engage with the necessary scientific gaze of objectivity, of being unable to participate in the discourses of standardised test scores and diagnostic labels (and other forms of discursive authority mobilised by professionals in the field of education and medicine) – parents are often expected to comply with professional judgement rather than collaborate on care plans for their children. And while these practices of marginalisation are by no means the experience of all parent-carers, it certainly appears to be widespread and routine.

However, there is a growing corpus of empirical work which suggests that parents are an excellent source of information on language development, memory, cognitive and motor skills.[25] Jinnah and Stoneman note that parents know their children and the rich array of strategies they use to teach and manage their children, but are never asked by providers to assist in any practices of problem solving.[26] Indeed parents themselves believe their own lived expertise yields useful information, and Fiks et al. have suggested that paediatric medics would benefit from training in shared decision-making.[27] Moreover, the literature suggests that parents are often best placed to notice small changes in developmental progress and have awareness of how services might be delivered more effectively for their child.[28]

Here we are interested in the space occupied between these two positions, noting that there appears to be a contradiction in the way that parental expertise is valued by the various apparatuses of the state with which they come into contact. It appears that while their forms of expertise may be frequently reduced to walk-on status when they engage with health and education professionals, this is not the case for their potential appropriateness as authorities of the caring regimes measured by the DLA form. In the realm of welfare suitability, of being able to provide an authoritative account both of their caring regime and of the variety of challenges that beset their child's everyday life, parents who have histories of exclusion are here constituted as those with the appropriate forms of expertise upon which judgements can be made on the suitability of a DLA award. Gone are the problems of failing to engage with labelling terminology, treatment regimes or objectivity. For this particular event, parents are adjudged sufficiently knowledgeable and responsible in accounting for their child's progress.

Amaze and the DLA Project

Swain et al. have suggested that 'disabling barriers' are useful for thinking about the mechanisms by which people are excluded from full participation in all aspects of civic life.[29] Being mindful of this, we spoke to a range of parents about their experiences with the children's DLA form, and their relations with a Brighton-based community project that seeks to support their successful completion of the form. Amaze is a registered charity active in the Brighton and Hove area. Its purpose is to inform, support and empower parents of children with disabilities and special needs. Central to the ethos of the organisation is a desire for parents' voices to be heard and to build their confidence and resilience so that they can support their children to lead happy and integrated lives. The organisation is parent-led and works with parent-carers of children with any additional needs aged 0 to 19 years. Amaze runs a number of services and projects, including their DLA Project.

The Amaze DLA Project aims to tackle poverty and social exclusion. It aims to maximise take-up of disability-related benefits amongst families with disabled children in Brighton and Hove, by providing a trained volunteer to support parent-carers to complete successful DLA applications. The DLA Project works with parents of children with a range of special needs, including challenging behaviour, mobility problems, visual and hearing problems, and moderate and severe learning difficulties. Between February and May 2012, 17 semi-structured interviews were carried out with a range of stakeholders relevant to the project. These included the project coordinator, three volunteer project workers and 13 parent-carers who had recently used the DLA Project. The children of parent participants had been diagnosed with a range of physical, learning and mental health disabilities, including cardiomyopathy, type 3 Ehlers–Danlos syndrome, autism and Down's syndrome.

The emotional challenge of the DLA form

For Star, boundary objects act as a means of translation and a tool for managing coherence across intersecting worlds, and they are useful as an analytic framework to understand information, lived experience and infrastructure.[30] They also tend to form the boundaries between groups that have the effect of shaping what can be known by one group about the other. Understanding the children's DLA form as a boundary object fulfils these properties but the experiences of our parents suggests that it tends toward a variety of other functions. It is our contention that the impact of this 'form as boundary object' calls to mind Swain et al.'s notion of disabling barriers. That is, the form itself constitutes a mechanism by which the families of children with complex needs are excluded from full participation in all aspects of civic life.

Banks and Lawrence note that the DLA form can leave carers feeling demoralised and frustrated.[31] In our conversations a number of people found the form very distressing and as such struggled not only to complete it but to engage with it at all. Many were loathed to reapply due to the stress of a process that they frequently found degrading and humiliating. The parents described the process of completing the form as 'hideous', 'really hard' and 'painful'. Most people found that completing the form was not just time-consuming and technically challenging, but highly distressing too.

> So it is really hard, and you're really dwelling on the fact that they're struggling and it's a really difficult situation, which you know, so, so it is hard. (Nicola, volunteer)

> I think that would just have been like, and it's, it's quite a painful process, you know, even telling you ... Those forms are so negative. (Danielle, parent)

> With Lucy, it was emotionally hideous to do, really hideous to document it. (Karen, parent)

The practice of writing down in great detail their children's difficulties – what their children could not do and where they struggled or failed – had a tremendous impact on parents and put many off from completing the form. There is no place on the form to think about the positive aspects of their child's life or their strengths and capacities. The 41-page trudge through their children's suffering and failings was reported to be a gruesome process that caused considerable distress by forcing the parent to focus on and elaborate in great detail just how difficult their child's life was, and how difficult their life was. For some it brought back feelings of profound anguish that they had worked hard not to dwell on. It forced parents, who had determined to focus on the positives, to rotate this stance and focus solely on their children's failings. We therefore argue that the emotional impact of this form should not be underestimated.

The technical challenges of the DLA form

There has been substantial criticism of the DLA form due to its complexity of structure, the high likelihood of making errors during application, and significant under-application, particularly amongst those most in need. Steyn et al. found that children in disadvantaged families are less likely to apply for and receive DLA.[32] Indeed the fact that 97.3 per cent of claimants found the form difficult to complete may account for the fact that 42.9 per cent of applicants initially turned down were subsequently given awards.[33] The form is an emotional challenge but it is also a technical challenge which, at 41 pages, makes it a daunting prospect for parents who are routinely pushed to their limits in terms of the energy and time that they have to devote to issues other than essential everyday survival.

A long and technically difficult form is an extreme challenge in these circumstances, and the emotional trauma of its completion, in conjunction with the technical difficulty, is likely to contribute both to the low number of applications and the large number of eligible families who are rejected. The vast majority of our parents noted, regardless of their literacy or educational qualifications, that the form was prohibitively complex.

> I would have to go through a long process. Because I would have just misunderstood the questions and just write something completely different to what they are asking, then I end up in a situation where they say no, we're not going to give it to you. (Jayne, parent)

> I've got a BA and I've got an MA, and I couldn't do it, I just couldn't do it. I'm articulate, I'm educated, I should be able to. (Kathy, parent)

> If I were to have to sit down and do those forms myself, I probably wouldn't have been as detailed, and I would have been very depressed by the end of it and it's very difficult, because you, because you know that the DLA are looking for certain words, certain things that trigger, like a points system, and [Amaze helper] knows all that. (Stacie, parent)

The experiences of the parents interviewed suggest that this boundary object does more than shape knowledge and act as a tool of translation across intersecting worlds; it can have the properties of an often profound emotional and technical challenge, affecting the people on one side of the translational divide in quite a profound manner. Based on the experiences of the parents we spoke to, the form *acts as a barrier* to gaining the awards that are so essential for parents and families. In so doing, it has the capacity to reproduce and perpetuate the systematic inequalities experienced by those with children with complex needs.

Earlier we outlined a potential paradox in parents being expected to provide the required expertise in order to ascertain appropriate welfare support while having their expertise routinely rejected, marginalised and discounted in the realms of medicine and education. However, while parental input is central to the DLA process, it is our contention that the nature of the form means that parents are in this instance party to a further form of marginalisation and disempowerment. Whereas in medicine and health it is the specialised technical discourses, procedures and practices of the professionals which wittingly or unwittingly facilitate this marginalisation, in the domain of welfare it is the structure of the boundary object itself. Both forms of activity exclude parental expertise: one through the technical/emotional challenge of integrating into the world of professionals and their privileged discourses, the other through the technical/emotional challenges of being nominated as 'expert' in a process with which they have no meaningful expertise. This is not to say that parent-carers do not know their children's difficulties or cannot describe their own caring regimes. Rather, they are not able to engage with this particular boundary object. Those who require DLA support and are entitled to it are disadvantaged in a number of ways. They find themselves party to a very considerable technical challenge – for some, a hideous 41-page emotional trial – and have to provide accounts of their caring regime with little understanding of the criteria upon which judgements will be made. For those without support this form can take days or weeks to complete, as parents entrained into passive walk-on roles in the recording of their lived experiences find themselves unsupported in this new arena of parental 'empowerment'.

In 2015 the governmental administration of welfare payments, indeed of any form of state dependency, is dominated by an ethos of suspicion.[34] Neoliberal strategies of government are dependent on devices that create individuals who do not need to be governed and supported but who can govern themselves.[35] In the neoliberal age there is a premium on the need to govern better through governing less, to produce an emergent subject who does not need to be governed by others but embodies a citizenship that is active and individualistic rather than passive and dependent.[36,37] In this culture, dependency has come to be understood as inimical to human dignity and self-determination, the prime virtue of the neoliberal subject.

Dean notes that anti-dependency is a vocabulary of rule that conditions and is conditioned by the way that we govern ourselves and others.[38] It is not only symbolic of social relations but also allows practices and programmes to operate in certain ways. In the neoliberal age, social insurance as a principle of social solidarity has given way to a privatisation of risk management. Here, insurance against the future possibilities of unemployment, ill health, old age, disability and the like becomes a private obligation.[39] Neoliberal government deploys indirect means for the surveillance and regulation of that agency whereby specific technologies, such as the DLA form, regulate how subjects can be known and hence acted upon.[40] Knowing an object such that it can be governed is more than a speculative activity; it requires procedures of notation such that they can be rendered in a particular conceptual form. The dependency that is so anathema to the neoliberal subject is carefully policed by a range of boundary objects between citizens and the state, and the necessity to police dependency ensures that these boundary objects carefully guard against the risk of inappropriate claims and the possibility of 'false positives' even if 'true negatives' are sacrificed in the process.

And so boundary objects can be said to do things. They impact upon people, frustrate them; they make the process of translation technically difficult and emotionally draining, and leave behind a residue on those who have engaged with it. The boundary object not only enables the translation of information, to allow a consensus to develop between intersecting worlds; it can also disable this process of translation, to make the conversion of information more difficult and more challenging. It acts not just as a means of translation but as a means of non-translation, not just to develop coherence but to develop incoherence between intersecting worlds, to frustrate consensus, to enable a means to 'not know'.

The DLA form as validation

The receipt of an award has a symbolic significance that can fundamentally resonate with the identity of the applicant as a parent. This was felt to be profoundly important to the many parents who had experienced long periods of uncertainty regarding the way that they are parenting their child with additional needs.

> So getting the highest level of DLA for her was a massive validation that she was really ill. And so actually getting that money, it was like somebody's recognising this. (Ann, parent)

> So, for many parents, getting the DLA, it is often the first time they get a real acknowledgment that they *are* doing stuff that's extra and different and more for their child. And that's really important when what they've

experienced, for years and years, might have been, 'You're an over-anxious parent,' you know, 'You're worrying too much. There's nothing really the matter; he'll soon shape up.' (Lizzie, manager)

Parents talked about the importance of their award in terms of validating their understanding of their child's difficulties, when very often they had felt pathologised by other agencies. For a number of parents, their suffering, trauma and difficulties were understood and validated by their receipt of the award. It validated their approach as parents in the various battles they faced to get their child the support they needed. Moreover, a successful award was seen to recognise the extra work they had been doing, often in the face of hints and accusations of overbearing parental concern. A successful award had genuine symbolic significance above and beyond the financial.

To reduce *en masse* the prospects of obtaining an award not only guards against dependency but also guards against parents being able to experience a validation of the life events, caring regimes and identities that necessarily precede their coming to understand themselves as deserving of forms of state dependence. Thus parents who have extra workloads, social isolation, financial strain, and demeaning encounters with professionals (and who would benefit from respite, support and dependency) are constrained from coming to understand themselves and the challenges they face in terms of the pressures they are under.[41,42]

The impact of the Amaze DLA Project

Banks and Lawrence note that DLA claimants are more successful if they receive professional or informed help with their application.[43] The Amaze DLA Project, through using a range of strategies to minimise the emotional and technical difficulty of the form, had a profound effect not only on the impact of the form on the parents but on their likelihood of receiving an award too.

And we just, we just went through it and I, I, well then I began to realise well actually, he teased it all out. He then gave it language. He was then able to link the things that I couldn't do; he could make links that I just couldn't see. (Sally, parent)

So yeah, so [Amaze helper] holding my hand, doing that was, she just let me talk, she basically put it on the computer, took it off, redid it all, and she went to the school and asked their views on Bobby as well. That was quite difficult because they put a lot of stuff about biting and kicking and stuff like that, but then I suppose I do see him a bit rose-tinted. (Joan, parent)

I'd probably feel even more isolated. I certainly would be worried, I would be worrying now about whether the forms that I'd filled in and sent off were going to be read properly, and that I was going to get the award that I need, whereas at the moment, because [Amaze helper] has taken care of that, I'm not worried about it at all. So she's taken one thing away from me that I don't have to worry about. (Roberta, parent)

Yes, because when [Amaze helper] filled in the form she said, 'But you can't do that, can you?' And she made me bring out things that I hadn't really thought about. (Rosanna, parent)

Boundary objects like the DLA form have the capacity to 'do things'. They have the capacity not only to impact upon people by confusing or by making possible an experience that is emotionally punishing, by facilitating or frustrating the process of translation, by squeezing and shaping what can be known or not known; they can also impact upon the social relational infrastructure of communities. As a direct result of the properties of the DLA form as a boundary object, a community organisation has developed a funded service, with paid workers, a coordinator, training regimes, volunteers, practices and procedures, and an office space. The work of the Amaze DLA Project reconfigures the activity of this particular boundary object. They ameliorate the impact of the form and facilitate the process of translation through reducing the form's formidable capacity to render carers' lives 'unknowable'. In so doing, the work of this organisation acts to denature a neoliberal technology that excludes parents. The work of such a service fundamentally alters the properties of the form as a boundary object. In so doing they contribute a resistance to the patrolling of dependency that would otherwise lead to a great many parent-carers not getting money that they desperately need and are entitled to. For a more detailed account of the ways in which Amaze fulfils this function see Walker and Streatfield.[44]

Concluding thoughts

This chapter accounts for the children's DLA form as one of Swain's 'disabling barriers', but also as an example of Star and Griesemer's 'boundary object', to reflect on a technology that has the potential impact of excluding many families from full participation in all aspects of civic life.[45,46] There is a disjunct between the ways in which parents are expected to have the very considerable expertise necessary to complete a technically challenging 41-page assessment form alone, but not to have sufficient expertise when liaising with the institutions that govern their children's health and education. This is explained through understanding the DLA form not only as a boundary object but also as one of a number of specific technologies that regulate how neoliberal subjects can be known and acted upon.

The dependency that is so inimical to the neoliberal subject is, in this context, carefully and effectively policed by the children's DLA form. Hence the 97.3 per cent of carers who find it 'difficult to complete', the 31 per cent of eligible children who don't apply, and the 42.9 per cent of eligible applicants who do apply but are initially turned down.[47] Just as Fassin and d'Halluin note that the deployment of the medical certificate in policing the climate of suspicion is central to asylum-seekers, the DLA form enacts a similar purpose in the arena of UK welfare support. In so doing it guards against the dangers both of dependency and a cynical misappropriation of public funds. However, such regimes of practice contribute to the desolation and distress of the many parent-carers struggling with financial strain following this practice of exclusion. The Amaze DLA Project is one example of an organisation that acts to disrupt this practice and, in so doing, contributes to a rebalancing of the relationship between policing dependency and supporting those in need.

Endnotes

1. Banks, P. & Lawrence, M. (2005). Transparent or opaque? Disabled people in Scotland describe their experiences of applying for disability living allowance. *Journal of Social Work*, 5 (3) 299–317.
2. Walker, C. & Streatfield, J. (2012). *The Amaze disability Living Allowance Project and the Experiences of the Parents who Use the Service*. Brighton: University of Brighton School of Applied Social Science.
3. Shahtahmasebi, S., Emerson, E., Berridge, D. & Lancaster, G. (2010). A longitudinal analysis of poverty among families supporting a child with a disability. *International Journal on Disability and Human Development*, 9 (1) 65–75.
4. Olsson, M. B. & Hwang, C. P. (2006). Well-being, involvement in paid work and division of child-care in parents of children with intellectual disabilities in Sweden. *Journal of Intellectual Disability Research*, 50 (12) 963–969.
5. Emerson, E. (2003). Mothers of children and adolescents with intellectual disability: Social and economic situation, mental health status, and the self-assessed social and psychological impact of the child's difficulties. *Journal of Intellectual Disability Research*, 47 (4/5) 385–399.

6. Steyn, B. J., Schneider, J. & McArdle, P. (2002). The role of Disability Living Allowance in the management of attention-deficit/hyperactivity disorder. *Child: Care, health & development*, 28 (6) 523–527.
7. Star, S. L. (2010). This is not a boundary object: Reflections on the origin of a concept. *Science, Technology & Human Values*, 35 (5) 601–617.
8. Star, S. L. & Griesemer, J. R. (1989). Institutional ecology: 'Translations' and boundary objects: Amateurs and professionals in Berkeley's Museum of Vertebrate Zoology, 1907–39. *Social Studies of Science*, 19 (3) 387–420.
9. Langan, M. (1998). *Welfare: Needs, rights and risks*. London: Routledge.
10. Fassin, D. & d'Halluin, E. (2005). The truth from the body: Medical certificates as ultimate evidence for asylum seekers. *American Anthropologist*, 107 (4) 597–608.
11. Valle, J. W. & Aponte, E. (2002). IDEA and collaboration: A Bakhtinian perspective on parent and professional discourse. *Journal of Learning Disabilities*, 35, 469–479.
12. Das, V. (2007). Commentary: Trauma and testimony: Between law and discipline. *ETHOS*, 35 (3) 330–335.
13. Berg, M. (1997). Of forms, containers and the electronic medical record: Some tools for a sociology of the formal. *Science, Technology & Human Values*, 22 (4) 403–433.
14. Star, 2010. See note 7.
15. Fassin & d'Halluin, 2005. See note 10.
16. Das, 2007. See note 12.
17. Gill, R. (2008). Culture and subjectivity in neoliberal and postfeminist times. *Subjectivity*, 25, 432–445.
18. Valle & Aponte, 2002. See note 11.
19. Foucault, M. (1980). *Power/Knowledge: Selected interviews and other writings 1972–1977*. New York: Pantheon.
20. Reid, K. R. & Valle, J. W. (2004). The discursive practice of learning disability: Implications for instruction and parent-school relations. *Journal of Learning Disabilities*, 37 (6) 466–481.
21. Moen, Ø. L., Hall-Lord, M. L. & Hedelin, B. (2011). Contending and adapting every day: Norwegian parents' lived experiences of having a child with ADHD. *Journal of Family Nursing*, 17, 441.
22. Woodcock, J. & Tregaskis, C. (2008). Understanding structural and communication barriers to ordinary life for families with disabled children: A combined social work and social model of disability analysis. *British Journal of Social Work*, 38, 55–71.
23. dosReis, S., Barksdale, C. L., Sherman, A., Maloney, K. & Charach, A. (2010). Stigmatizing experiences of parents of children with a new diagnosis of ADHD. *Psychiatric Services*, 61 (8) 811.
24. Walker & Streatfield, 2012. See note 2; Urey, J. R. & Viar, V. (1990). Use of mental health and support services among families of children with disabilities: Discrepant views of parents and paediatricians. *Mental Handicap Research*, 3 (1) 81–88.
25. Dewey, D. D., Crawford, S. G. & Kaplan, B. J. (2003). Clinical importance of parent ratings of everyday cognitive abilities in children with learning and attention problems. *Journal of Learning Disabilities*, 36, 87.
26. Jinnah, H. A. & Stoneman, Z. (2008). Parents' experiences in seeking child care for school age children with disabilities: Where does the system break down? *Children and Youth Services Review*, 30, 967–977.
27. Fiks, A., Hughes, C. C., Gafen, A., Guevara, J. P. & Barg, F. K. (2011). Contrasting parents' and paediatricians' perspectives on shared decision making in ADHD. *Pediatrics*, 127, e188–e196.
28. Woodcock & Tregaskis, 2008. See note 22.

29. Swain, J., Finkelstein, V., French, S. & Oliver, M. (2004). *Disabling Barriers: Enabling environments* (2nd edition). London: Sage.
30. Star, 2010. See note 7.
31. Banks & Lawrence, 2005. See note 1.
32. Steyn et al., 2002. See note 6.
33. Banks & Lawrence, 2005. See note 1.
34. Fassin & d'Halluin, 2005. See note 10; Das, 2007. See note 12.
35. Rose, N. (1996). Governing 'advanced' liberal democracies. In A. Barry, T. Osborne & N. Rose (Eds). *Foucault and Political Reason: Liberalism, neoliberalism and rationalities of government* (pp. 37–64). Chicago: University of Chicago Press.
36. Terkelsen, T. B. (2009). Transforming subjectivities in psychiatric care. *Subjectivity*, 27, 195–216.
37. Miller, P. & Rose, N. (2008). *Governing the Present*. Cambridge: Polity Press.
38. Dean, M. (1999). *Governmentality: Power and rule in modern society*. Los Angeles, CA: Sage.
39. Rose, 1996. See note 35.
40. Dean, 1999. See note 38.
41. Kobayashi, T., Inagaki, M. & Kaga, M. (2011). Professional caregiver's view on mental health in parents of children with developmental disabilities: A nationwide study of institutions and consultation centres in Japan. *ISRN Pediatrics*, 121898.
42. Mullins, L. L., Aniol, K., Boyd, M. L., Page, M. C. & Chaney, J. M. (2002). The influence of respite care on psychological distress in parents of children with developmental disabilities: A longitudinal study. *Children's Services: Social policy, research and practice*, 5 (2) 123–138.
43. Banks & Lawrence, 2005. See note 1.
44. Walker & Streatfield, 2012. See note 2.
45. Swain et al., 2004. See note 29.
46. Star & Griesemer, 1989. See note 8.
47. Banks & Lawrence, 2005. See note 1.

About the contributors

Abigail Bray

Dr Abigail Bray is a senior research consultant for the School of Indigenous Studies at the University of Western Australia. She has published books and newspaper, magazine and academic journal articles on adolescent mental health, gender, sexuality and violence and children's rights. She is an inaugural inductee in the UN-sponsored WA Women's Hall of Fame and has presented papers at the House of Lords in the UK, at parliament in Australia and at The Hague, among other places.

Peter R. Breggin, MD

Peter R. Breggin, MD, is known as the 'conscience of psychiatry' for his decades of reform work. He has authored dozens of articles and more than 20 books, including *Brain-disabling Treatments in Psychiatry*, *Psychiatric Drug Withdrawal*, and *Guilt, Shame and Anxiety: Understanding and overcoming negative emotions*. See www.breggin.com

Melissa Burkett

Melissa holds a BA in psychology and criminology and a first class honours degree in criminology and justice. Her PhD explores young peoples' negotiations of sexualised culture and pornography. She has published academic work broadly in the areas of gender and sexuality with a key focus on the contemporary context of sexualisation, neoliberalism and post-feminism. In her (limited) spare time she enjoys reading, gardening, walking her dog and attempting to teach herself how to play guitar.

Carmen Cubillo

Carmen Cubillo is a founding member of the Australian Indigenous Psychologists Association and a former Convenor of the Australian Psychological Society Interest Group Aboriginal and Torres Strait Islander Peoples and Psychology. Carmen's doctoral research project focuses on measuring changes in observed parent–child interaction between Indigenous and non-Indigenous parents within the Let's Start Exploring Together Program in the Northern Territory. She is a full member of the Australian College of Clinical Psychologists. Carmen is also a placement co-ordinator for clinical master's students and the co-ordinator of play therapy courses at Charles Darwin University. Carmen's current areas of expertise are transcultural counselling, attachment problems, and psychotherapy with children and adolescents. Carmen's research is dedicated to shedding light on the underlying issues of Aboriginal health and wellbeing and contributing to improving practice and research with Aboriginal communities.

Rudi Dallos

Rudi Dallos is Professor and Research Director on the D.Clin. Psychology training programme at the University of Plymouth. He has developed an orientation to working with families – Attachment Narrative Therapy – and offers training and consultation in this model. He has written several books including *Attachment Narrative Therapy*, *Formulation in Psychotherapy and Counselling* and *An Introduction to Family Therapy*. He is currently developing research programmes to explore the links between family dynamics, attachment and constructions of autism and psychosis.

Pat Dudgeon

Professor Pat Dudgeon is from the Bardi people of the Kimberley in Western Australia. She is an Aboriginal psychologist and has made outstanding contributions to Indigenous psychology and higher education. She has undertaken much work and many publications in this area and is considered one of the 'founding' people in Indigenous psychology. Pat was inaugural Chair of the Australian Indigenous Psychologists Association. Pat is a Commissioner for the Australian National Mental Health Commission. Among numerous positions, Pat is Research Professor and Project Leader, ARC Discovery Indigenous Grant, the School of Indigenous Studies, University of Western Australia; Chief Investigator on NHMRC Centre for Research Excellence in Aboriginal Health and Wellbeing; Honorary Research Fellow, Telethon Institute for Child Health Research, University of Western Australia; and Project Leader, the National Empowerment Project. She is actively involved with the Aboriginal community, having an ongoing commitment to social justice for Indigenous people. Pat has participated in numerous state and national committees, councils, task groups and community service activities.

Adele Gladman

Adele Gladman left legal practice in 2000 to lead on a UK Home Office research and development pilot addressing issues of child sexual exploitation (CSE). She has since delivered safeguarding-children work across the UK, including developing policies and procedures, assisting legal services, conducting independent investigations and audits, and helping organisations to attain best practice standards. Adele continues to work closely with victims of CSE, and their families.

Laura Golding

Dr Laura Golding is a clinical psychologist and Academic Director of the University of Liverpool's Doctorate in Clinical Psychology. She has worked with adults with learning disabilities throughout much of her career. She has published research in the field of learning disabilities as well as on supervision and continuing professional development, and is Co-editor of *Continuing Professional Development for Clinical Psychologists: A practical handbook* (BPS Blackwell, 2006).

Dan Goodley

Dan Goodley is Professor of Disability Studies at the University of Sheffield. He is author of a number of texts including *Disability Studies* (Sage, 2010) and *Dis/ability Studies* (Routledge, 2014). His work focuses on theorising and contesting the dual processes of ableism and disableism.

Carl Harris

Carl Harris is a 51-year-old NHS clinical psychologist with 20 years' experience of working with children and families in community settings. He has a BA in political economy and an MPhil in political theory and philosophy. Between 2001 and 2006 he worked in community regeneration in Birmingham, UK.

Orly Klein

Orly Klein is a senior lecturer in psychology at the University of Brighton. She has published in the field of reality and makeover television, and now specialises in critical parental studies, currently focusing on challenging the denigration of women who bottle feed.

Carolyn McQueen

Dr Carolyn McQueen is a shaman and clinical psychologist. She has worked in Young Offender Institutions and now specialises in work with foster families and looked-after children. With Craig Newnes she helped create the Staffordshire Doctorate in Clinical Psychology based at Stoke, Keele and Shropshire.

Craig Newnes

Craig Newnes is a consulting critical psychologist, editor and author. He has published numerous book chapters and academic articles and is Editor of the *Journal of Critical Psychology, Counselling and Psychotherapy.* He was, for 19 years, the Editor of *Clinical Psychology Forum* (the in-house practice journal of the Division of Clinical Psychology of the British Psychological Society) and Director of Psychological Therapies for Shropshire's Community and Mental Health Services Trust. He is ex-Chair of the Psychotherapy Section of the BPS.

He has edited five books and is Commissioning Editor for six further volumes in the Critical Psychology Division from PCCS Books. In 2014 he authored *Clinical Psychology: A critical examination* as part of the PCCS Critical Examination series for which he is also Commissioning Editor. His most recent volume is *Inscription, Diagnosis and Deception in the Mental Health Industry: How Psy governs us all* (Palgrave Macmillan, 2015). He is a visiting lecturer at Queen's University, Belfast, and Murdoch University, Fremantle, and an Honorary Lecturer at 11 UK universities. He continues to lecture and write and in 2005 received the CCHR Award in Human Rights for 20 years of speaking out about the Psy complex.

Katherine Runswick-Cole

Katherine Runswick-Cole is Senior Research Fellow in Disability Studies and Psychology at Manchester Metropolitan University. She locates her work in the field of critical disability studies.

Carl Walker

Carl Walker is a critical community psychologist from the University of Brighton. His interests include informal therapeutic practices, the manufacturing of suffering through the everyday application of local and national debt industries, and community university partnerships. He also likes cycling.

Name Index

A
Adams, M. 63
Allen, G. 87
Allison, H. 73
Anderson, I. 53
Aponte, E. 232, 234
Ariès, P. 165
Atkinson, J. 73, 74
Aziz, M. 196

B
Bailey, R. 38
Baldwin, S. 190
Banks, P. 237, 241
Barnhill, L. 151
Bateson, G. (1904–1980) 217, 219
Bender, L. 185
Bennett, A. 212
Bennett, M. 61, 62
Berg, M. 232
Bernier, A. 115
Bettelheim, B. (1903–1990) 16
Bhabha, H. 54
Biederman, J. 19, 152
Bini, L. 185
Biskup P. 55
Bogdan, R. 163
Booth, C. 21
Bowlby, J. (1907–1990) 16, 114, 219, 225, 228
Boyle, D. 20
Breggin, P. 182
Bronfenbrenner, U. (1917–2005) 83
Broome, R. 55
Brown, G. 38
Brown, G.W. 108, 117
Bruch, H. 217
Byng-Hall, J. 225

C
Cameron, D. 37, 38
Carlson, L. 163
Castellanos, F.X. 148

Chritcher, C. 36
Cohen, D. 186
Coulter, C. 221–224, 227
Cummings, B. 68

D
Danet, M. 115
Darwin, C. (1809–1882) 14
Das, V. 233
Dean, M. 239
deMause, L. 11, 18
d'Halluin, E. 232, 233, 243
Diaz, C. 193
Dickens, C. (1812–1870) 10
Dineen, T. 24
dosReis, S. 234
Duchenne, G.B.C. 183
Dudgeon, P. 74, 75
Duren, J. 67
Duschinsky, R. 34, 36, 45
Dyer, M. 68

E
Egan, D. 34, 40, 44
Engels, F. (1820–1895) 12
Erikson, E. 16

F
Fassin, D. 232, 233, 243
Fiks, A. 235
Findling, R. 19
Fischer, N. 44
Foucault, M. (1926–1984) 15, 16, 21, 36, 37, 206, 213
Freud, A. (1895–1982) 16
Freud, S. (1856–1939) 42
Frith, U. 20, 22

G
Garbarino, J. 40
Gale, J. 39
Gesell, A. (1880–1961) 14, 185

Gonick, M. 43
Goodman, H. 85
Gottstein, J. 156
Griesemer, J.R. 232, 242
Gualtieri, C. 151

H
Haebich, A. 52
Haig-Brown, C. 57
Hall, S. 43
Hamann, S. 74
Harper, S. 58
Haraldsdóttir, F. 177
Havens, R. (1941–2013) 28
Hawkes, G. 34, 40, 44
Henson, B. 39
Herman, R.C. 191
Hippocrates 214
Howard, J. 65
Howlin, P. 21, 22
Hseih, M-O. 116
Hughes, D.A. 209

J
Jackson, E. 134
Jackson, S. 37
Jacobs, M.D. 59, 62
James, A. 165
James, M. 182
Jenkins, P. 36
Jinnah, H.A. 235
Jones, Y. 190

K
Kanner, L. 20, 218
Keating, P. 52, 64
Keller, H. 69
Kelly, K. 74
Kincaid, J. 41
Klein, M. 16
Kraepelin, E. (1856–1926) 18

L
Laing, R.D. 219
Lambert, N. 148
Langan, M. 232
Larkin, P. (1922–1985) 212
Lawrence, M. 237, 241
Leiberman, J. 153
LeRoy, J.B. 183
Leung, P. 116
Levarch, M. 64

Levine, K. 116
Lima, N.N.R. 190
Lowe, M.E. 111
Lupton, D. 35

M
Macquarie, L. 65
Marx, K. (1818–1883) 12, 215
Maynard, C. 67
McClelland, R.J. 182
McClement, S.E. 111, 112
McGrath, A. 52
McHoul, A. 224
McKenzie, J.A. 175
McKenzie, L. 90
Mersey, J.C. 98
Miljkovitch, R. 115
Miller, A. 16
Mooney, A. 109
Mills, S. 50
Mooney, A. 109
Moran, P. 108, 117
Moreno, C. 152
Moreton-Robinson, A. 53, 56

N
Nelson, A. 73
Nelson, M. 107

P
Papadopoulos, L. 38
Pearce, J. 134
Peeters, L. 74, 75
Pipher, M. 43
Point, G. 59
Proal, E. 148
Prout, J. 165

R
Rapley, M. 28, 178, 221–224, 227
Renaud, A. 59
Rey, J.M. 186
Reynolds, H. 55
Roberts, E. 19
Robinson, K.H. 37
Roger of Salerno 183
Rose, N. 14, 42, 48
Rowe, D. 17
Rowley, C. 55
Rowling, J.K. 105, 118
Ryan, S. 173, 174
Rudd, K. 38, 52

Rutter, M. 21

S

Sament, S. 182
Schmideberg, M. 16
Scott, S. 37
Shaw, C. 183
Shorter, E. 192
Spencer, T. 152
Stanley Hall, G. 14
Stanner, W.E.H. 55
Star, S.L. 231, 233, 242
Staub, E. 182
Stein, D. 17
Steyn, B.J. 237
Stoneman, Z. 235
Stroup, T. 153
Sully, J. 14
Swain, J. 235, 242
Swanson, J. 148
Symonds, C.P. 182

T

Tankard Reist, M. 39
Taylor, S.J. 163
Tucker, M. 68
Tuhiwai Smith, L. 53, 56

V

Valle, J.W. 232, 234

W

Walker, R. 74
Walter, G. 186
Wearing, G. 106
Webb, S. 85
Wilens, T. 152
Willoughby, C.L. 187
Winnicott, D.W. (1896–1971) 16, 30

Z

Žižek, S. 171

Subject Index

A

Aboriginal and Torres Strait Islanders 51, 57, 63, 68-70, 75
accommodation 93, 95, 98, 122
adoption 67, 68
   Maori customs of 15
adverse effects
   brain atrophy 151
   and ADHD 148
   neuroleptic malignant syndrome 150-1, 186, 189
   of 'antipsychotic' drugs (tranquillisers) 153, 156
      tardive akathisia 150-1
      tardive dyskinesia 150-1, 159-60
      tardive dystonia 150
   of electroconvulsive therapy 182, 186, 188, 189, 192
      lobotomy-like indifference 150
   of parental separation 108
   of stimulant drugs (see amphetamines, methylphenidate)
      animal studies 149
      apathy 149-50, 153, 155, 156
      growth suppression 148
      MTA study 148, 150
      reduction of spontaneity 149, 155
'age of anxiety' 33
AIDS 8
alcohol 8, 57, 70, 122, 127, 133, 136, 166, 185
APA Report of the APA Task Force on the Sexualization of Girls 35, 36, 39
amphetamines 147-8
attachment 69, 70, 90, 102, 110-6, 129, 204-5, 208, 217-26
Attention Deficit Hyperactivity Disorder (ADHD) 1, 2, 19-23, 145-54, 165, 168, 213, 216, 224
   NIH Consensus Development Conference on, 148
   personal responsibility and, 149, 153
austerity 54, 82-100, 116, 204

Australia Institute 39
Australian Indigenous mental health movement 51, 68
autism 20-2, 146, 154, 167, 169, 187, 196, 213, 218, 228, 229, 236

B

Bailey Review 38
Bellevue Asylum 8
bereavement 102, 110-3, 118, 125, 206
Big Society, the 88, 167-8, 177
bipolar disorder 2, 10, 18, 19, 22, 145-6, 152, 154, 186-7
   increased inscription of, 2, 19, 22
blame
   of parents 212-228
   in relation to sexual exploitation 126, 133, 136
body image 35
boundary objects 231-44
Bringing Them Home: Report of the National Inquiry into the Separation of Aboriginal and Torres Strait Islander Children from their Families 51-74

C

caring regimes 233-41
child
   abuse 1, 122, 136, 140,
      psychiatric drugs as, 19
   labour 12, 32
   Psychotherapy Trust 22
   saving 43, 60
   Study Society 13
   welfare 25, 60, 66, 77, 132
child sexual exploitation (CSE)
   and emerging vulnerabilities 129-31
   and looked-after children 128-9, 134, 203
   as child abuse 122

as child protection issue 139-140
definition of, 122-3, 138
judging victims of, 133
professional responses to, 131-2
childhood
and the DLA form 168, 231, 233, 243
construction of, 10, 11, 33, 164-77, 207
definition of, 7-8, 27, 165, 184
innocence 9, 28, 33, 34, 37-46
myth of, 8-11, 27, 28
children
'learning-disabled', 162-177, 190, 191
Children's Crusade 11
citizenship 239
civil rights movement 68
class 11, 22, 42, 44, 60, 83, 92, 94, 98
working-, 11, 41, 44, 60, 92
middle-, 11, 16, 21, 40, 42, 44-6
family 59, 60, 61, 65, 92
unemployed, 21
Collective Shout 39
colonisation 53-6, 64, 69, 73, 75
genocidal, 73
psychological, 59
complex needs 86, 128, 231-8
Corporate Paedophilia 39
cortisol 92, 95
Crip Schools 174-5

D

death 13, 59, 61, 70
and ECT, 186
antipsychotics and, 152
of a partner 103, 110-3
of a 'learning-disabled' child 173-4
parental, 136
of child, parental responsibility for, 214
through drug misuse 148
dependency
and psychiatric diagnosis 153
in child exploitation 134
on state benefits 86, 232, 234, 239-43
policing of, 239-43
psychological, 153
deprivation 82, 92
diagnosis 17, 18, 19, 23, 28, 168-9, 217-218
ADHD, effects of, 147-9

advantages of, 145-6, 168, 220, 221
and ECT 189-90
and labelling 220-1
as a method of inscription 23, 25-6
harm caused by, 146, 152-4, 189, 191, 198
medical, 223
of autism 196, 218
of bipolar disorder 18
in children 19-20, 152
of depression 108
of 'learning disability' 168
politics of, 164
Diagnostic and Statistical Manual (DSM) 17, 18, 152, 159, 204, 213
disability
and lifespan 83
and vulnerability 126-8, 145
learning, 23, 162-77, 187, 190-1
rights 191
Living Allowance (DLA) 231-5
disadvantage/disadvantage
and ill health 52
in education and employment 70
of First Peoples in court 65
social/economic, 85-7, 89, 92, 153, 194, 231, 238
discourse
around care 206
biopolitical, 45, 46, 54, 60, 61, 219
of Australian nationhood 56
of inscription 22, 27
of neoliberal individualism 54
of sexualisation 34, 35, 37
professional, 23, 24, 41, 197, 223, 224, 228, 234, 239, 244
rights 24
scientific (scientistic), 14, 17, 164, 197, 213, 235
discrimination 70, 73, 173-4
displacement, forced 70
disqualification of parents' voices 232
divorce 15, 102-21, 206

E

Economic and Social Science Research Council 177
education 7, 9-12, 25, 35-8, 42, 45, 56, 59-71, 89, 108, 124, 132, 133, 135, 145, 162, 167, 170-7, 184, 234-5, 239, 243
Enjoyment of Sexualisation Scale 36

environment/environmental factors 2, 25, 26, 40, 43, 56, 70, 72, 82, 87, 90-3, 116, 145, 154, 171, 205-8, 217
'estatism' 90
eugenics 60, 66-7, 178

F

fathers
   estrangement from, 113
   First Peoples, 51, 59, 70, 72
   single-parent, 103, 115
forgiveness 212, 214
Fort Bragg Demonstration Project 23-4
foster
   parents/carers 2, 15, 125, 139, 205-10
   homes/care 67, 126, 204
   placements 124, 125

G

gaze, the 14, 21, 234
genocide 51, 53, 61, 65, 70, 74, 76
   Armenian, 12
   cultural, 57
   UN Convention Against, 65
Gingerbread 104, 105
Good Childhood Inquiry 37
governance 75, 171, 233
government
   and rights of children 13, 24, 25, 35, 37, 50, 62, 65, 70, 84-6, 89, 97, 122, 146, 170, 204, 233
governmentality 14, 24, 36
Grandmothers Against Removals (Gunnedah group) 50, 68
guilt 136, 212-4, 228

H

Hansel and Gretel 9
healing 51, 225
   First Peoples, 68-76
housing/council estates 82, 88, 90, 91, 92
human rights
   and Psy abuses 191
   of First Peoples 51, 58, 64, 74

I

illegal/illegality 60, 136
   of ECT 194-7
Imagine Chicago 26

indigenous child-rearing 69
inequality 25, 82, 83, 94
innocence (see childhood – innocence)
International Classification of Disease (ICD) 18, 213
Iraq 13, 24

K

Kids Free 2B Kids 39-40

L

legal aid 89
Letting Children Be Children: Stopping the sexualisation of children in Australia 38, 39

M

medical professionals 43, 234
mental health
   National Service Framework (NSF) for, 26
   services, child and adolescent (CAMHS), 7, 26, 123, 184, 204
   state systems of, 152
methylphenidate 147-9 (see also adverse effects – stimulant drugs)
monitoring (see also the gaze) 23, 45, 71, 93
   DLA claims 231
moral
   agendas 43
   behaviour 86
   crusade 60
   entrepreneur 37
   corruption of childhood 40, 43, 45
   danger to the child 42, 43
   narrative 87
   panics 37, 41, 42, 47, 62
   purity 33, 34, 37, 44, 46
   reading of childhood 35
   wellbeing 146, 154, 155, 156
mother/motherhood
   '-blaming' 217, 220
   First Peoples, 52, 57, 61, 62, 64, 66, 71
   as primary carer of children with 'learning disability' 170
   teenage, 15, 104, 106,
   single,
      and attachment 114
      and bereavement 110-1
      by choice 103

positives of, 110, 115–8
negatives of, 116–7
Mothers' Union 38
Mumsnet 38, 39

N

neighbourhood 90, 92, 93
neoliberal(ism) 37, 43, 45, 54, 83, 245
neuroleptic drugs (see adverse effects – antipsychotic drugs)
non-engagement 134–8

O

Oily Cart theatre company, The 176

P

parents/parenting/parenthood 17–28
adoptive, 216
and smacking 24–5
and stress 93, 94
as teamwork 113–4
communal, in First Peoples, 68–73
concerns about child mental health 18–19
consent to ECT 187
'double-', 111–3
involvement in service evaluation 26
models of responsibility 217–9
needs for support 17
non-biological, 15
poor quality, 123, 234
of 'learning-disabled' babies/children 166–7, 171, 173, 177, 184, 231, 232, 234, 236, 239
rights 39
termination of, 146
separation 84, 102, 103, 108–13, 116
single-/lone, 15, 90, 93, 102–21
widowed, 110–2
play 169–170, 175–7
'Politics of Suspicion' 233
Ponderosa 7
poverty 21, 25, 54, 60, 83–100, 102, 104, 106–9, 147, 194, 236
prostitute 44, 133
'prostitution', child 139
psychology
clinical, 1, 24
developmental, 14, 35
indigenous, 51, 74
positive, 208

power imbalance 26
Western, 76
psychosurgery as treatment for psychiatric disorders 155, 197
Put Britain Back on Her Feet 37

O

'Ophelia industry' 42–5
Other, the
evil, contaminated, 37, 42–5
deviant, 51

R

race 11, 42, 46, 145
white, Australia, 52, 74
white, middle-class 41, 42, 44
racism 54, 63, 71, 76, 194
Redfern Park Speech 52
relationships
abusive, 132–3, 140
ending of, 110, 111, 115, 123
family/parenting, 51, 69, 86, 110, 111
healthy, 95, 124, 127,
parent–child, 11, 14, 110, 115, 208
problems with social, 20
re-alignment of, 16
sexual, 9, 117, 122–4, 138, 185 (see also child sexual exploitation)
social, 73
resilience 70–5, 102, 109, 110, 112, 116–7, 236
resources 45, 82, 91–5, 123, 133, 137, 175, 204
Rotherham 123, 129, 130, 141, 203
Home Office-funded research and development pilot 123, 129

S

self 54, 70, 114, 206, 210, 217, 219, 228
-determination 75–6, 149, 153, 239
-esteem 35, 43, 124, 153
inscription of, 14
SENCOs (Special Educational Needs Co-ordinators) 234
separation 84, 102–3, 108, 109–116, 171, 207
of First People children 51, 64, 68, 70, 74
sexualisation
constructing the crisis about, 34–6, 37, 38, 39, 44

Index 257

improper/proper, 33, 34, 36, 39
politics of/and policy towards, 36–40
Sexualising Behaviours Scale 36
sexuality 34, 37, 39–42, 44,–6, 63, 131
slavery 12, 27
social and cultural systems, levels of
    exo level 84, 87–9
    macro level 84–5
    meso level 84, 90–1
    micro level 84, 91, 93–4
social
    construction(ism) 33, 162–5, 209
    exclusion/excluded 86, 94, 236
    inclusion 91, 94
socioeconomic status 91 (see *also* disadvantage – social/economic)
spirituality 57, 75, 76, 195
stigma 90, 104–6, 116, 153
Stolen Generations 50, 56, 57, 63–5
Stress
    context of, 93, 222
    in childhood 93–5, 109
    in carers 208
    post-traumatic, 73, 74, 134
surveillance 36, 41–6, 170, 173

T

tardive dyskinesia/dystonia/akathisia (see adverse effects – of 'antipsychotic' drugs)
teacher(s) 2, 23, 43, 56, 61, 92, 94, 149, 167, 171, 175, 234
    'queer', 175
teenagers 7–9, 116, 184, 195 (see *also* mothers – teenage)
    and drug use 9
    depressed, 186
    radicalisation of, 8
trauma 52, 64, 67, 68, 70–6, 115, 128–9, 134–7, 140, 205, 207, 241
'Troubled Families' programme 85–6

U

United Nations Convention on the Rights of the Child 2, 24–6, 145, 191

V

violence 13, 25, 63, 83, 123, 128, 146, 173, 177, 194

and 'learning disabled' children 171–3
vulnerability (see also child sexual exploitation)
    'biological', 42–3
    created 45, 128, 138, 140
    stress model of, 222
    views of, 9, 33, 122–5

W

war 1, 8, 11–14, 27
welfare state 37, 86
wellbeing 22, 26, 33, 38, 42, 69, 71–2, 83, 94, 95, 106–9, 110, 114, 117
    social and emotional, 51, 53, 57, 63, 75–6, 114
    parental, 93
    moral, (see moral – wellbeing)
Widowed & Young 111

Y

Youthanasia 10